KV-462-461

Multiple Choice Questions on Surgical Diagnosis

A Companion to Hamilton Bailey's
Demonstrations of Physical Signs in Clinical Surgery, 18th Edition

R Visvanathan BM, FRCS
Consultant Surgeon, Bronglais General Hospital, Aberystwyth
Surgical Tutor, Royal College of Surgeons of England
Lately Honorary Senior Lecturer in Surgery and
Assistant Director to the Professorial Surgical Unit
The Medical College and Hospital of St Bartholomew, London

J S P Lumley MS, FRCS
Professor of Surgery and Honorary Consultant Surgeon
The Medical College and Hospital of St Bartholomew, London
Member of Council, Royal College of Surgeons of England
Past World President, International College of Surgeons

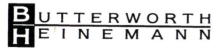

BUTTERWORTH
HEINEMANN

OXFORD AUCKLAND BOSTON JOHANNESBURG MELBOURNE NEW DELHI

Butterworth-Heinemann
Linacre House, Jordan Hill, Oxford OX2 8DP
225 Wildwood Avenue, Woburn, MA 01801-2041
A division of Reed Educational and Professional Publishing Ltd

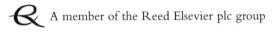 A member of the Reed Elsevier plc group

First published 2000

British Library Cataloguing in Publication Data
Visvanathan, R.
 MCQs on surgical diagnosis
 1 Diagnosis, Surgical – Examinations, questions, etc.
 I. Title   II. Lumley, J. S. P. (John Stuart Penton)
 617'.075'076

ISBN 0 7506 4730 2

Typeset by BC Typesetting, Keynsham, Bristol BS31 1NZ
Printed and bound in Great Britain by Biddles Ltd,
Guildford and King's Lynn

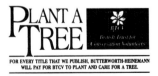

Contents

Preface

Multiple choice questions (MCQs) are a useful means of assessing the acquisition of a large amount of factual knowledge: for this reason they are commonly used in undergraduate and postgraduate medical examinations. They are of most value when based on a well-documented collection of information, be this a textbook or a detailed curriculum.

This text has been prepared to meet these requirements, the parent volume being Hamilton Bailey's *Demonstrations of Physical Signs in Clinical Surgery*, 18th edition, ed. J.S.P. Lumley, Oxford: Butterworth-Heinemann, ISBN 07506 16210. The answers and comments can be supplemented by reference to Hamilton Bailey's *Physical Signs*, which also contains an extensive selection of coloured illustrations of all common surgical conditions.

Introduction

The introduction of the MCQ over 50 years ago was the initial step in the progressive change from subjective to objective knowledge testing. Although the MCQ has been subjected to extensive study, modification and frequent criticism, it still provides one of the commonest forms of assessment in undergraduate and post-graduate medical education.

The strength of the MCQ is its ability to cover a wide range of topics in a consistent manner, while computer marking is economical on examiners' time and avoids a subjective element in the assessment. However, setting good MCQ questions is difficult, and candidates must be experienced in this examination format, so that they are examined on the content of the paper rather than skills in examination technique.

MCQ setting
MCQs should be produced by a panel including experts from all the relevant disciplines. The subjects and the depth of knowledge should be decided, together with the format of the examination; members of the panel should provide the first draft of questions within their areas of interest.

A common format is multiple True/False, with a stem and five options, any of which may be true or false. In matched pairs, another common variant, the candidate chooses the most appropriate answer from a given menu of possibilities.

Stems and options should be brief, using the minimum number of words, and instructions should be clear and simple, the language being appropriate to the verbal ability and requirements of the candidates. The questions must always be of some educational value. The distractors (wrong options) are the most exacting part of objective question composition, and the standard of an objective test is probably best assessed in terms of the quality of its distractors. They must all be plausible yet completely wrong. They should be in a parallel style to the correct responses and should not contain clues.

The wording of MCQs must avoid ambiguity and the choice can be challenging. Absolutes are rare in medicine and therefore words such as 'never' and 'always' are likely to be wrong and should be avoided. Similarly, anything 'may' or 'can' occur. Although 'commonly', 'usually' and 'frequently' are standard medical terminology, they carry potential hazards to a candidate, who might have obtained a different emphasis in his/her teaching; 'typical', 'characteristic' or 'recognized' are useful terminology.

Draft questions are circulated before the panel meets, when the value and limitations of questions are assessed, and inaccurate and irrelevant material excluded. Even the most experienced examiners will find that a panel will offer constructive criticism on the majority of their questions. Ideally, once the panel has assessed a series of questions, they should be pre-tested on a group of students, and the results analysed. It is desirable for questions to have been pre-tested on 300–400 students before they come into regular use in a qualifying examination.

The typical computer print-out of an examination provides not only a raw score and a rank order of candidates, but also indices on the discriminatory value and difficulty of each question. These factors must be reviewed after each use of a question, to ensure that it has appropriate educational value. A satisfactory bank of questions takes three to five years to build up and must be continuously updated and revised. Security of the bank is important but becomes less so as its size increases, since accurate knowledge of the whole bank is then equivalent to a satisfactory knowledge of the syllabus.

Answering MCQs
When undertaking an objective test, ensure that you have some preliminary experience of the expected form of assessment, and have sampled the style of questions used by your Examining Board. Read the instructions very carefully; marking is by computer and therefore no allowance is made for misunderstandings. Each question is intended to test a specific piece of knowledge. The wording has been chosen with this in mind and with great care. Good discriminants are difficult to formulate, so do not try to read hidden meanings or obscure facts into the answers. Beware, however, that common misconceptions are likely to be included.

Once you are sure of the format, read through the whole paper, marking on the computer form all the answers that you know to be correct. Avoid guessing as the negative marking is designed to penalize this practice. As these tests are of the 'power' rather than the 'speed' variety, there is usually plenty of time to go back over unanswered questions and 'play one's hunches' in areas that you are conversant with. It has been shown that this approach produces higher than random results. Mark the computer form rather than the question paper once you have decided on the answer, since although time is not usually a problem, transcribing a number of hundred marks in a hurry can introduce inaccuracies.

How to use this book

The MCQs are organized into sections which correspond to the chapters in Hamilton Bailey's *Demonstrations of Physical Signs in Clinical Surgery* (18th edition). The answers, with explanatory comments, are given in the second half of the book. The chapter and page(s) of the relevant text and illustrations in *Physical Signs* are given with each comment, so that the two books can be used together to incorporate all the available clinical material. We suggest that you attempt all questions in each section when revising the relevant chapters.

The Appendix contains a numerical list of selected MCQs from the book organized in an examination format, enabling you to gain the experience of working under timed conditions. Thirty MCQs constitute a 40-minute paper.

When self-marking, allocate one mark for each correct response and a negative mark for each incorrect response. The negative marking scoring system is to discourage guessing or random marking which in a true/false answer scenario could otherwise provide a false positive result. This would undermine the effectiveness of this form of assessment: negative marking encourages a disciplined and circumspect approach to the questions. These mock papers are intended to provide an assessment of your performance and highlight areas of deficiency. The MCQs in each section and the sections themselves follow the order of presentation in Hamilton Bailey. When a topic is addressed in different sections in Hamilton Bailey the questions on it are placed in the most appropriate section and the references cited in chronological order. The sections are independent of each other, allowing you to revise the chapters in your order of preference.

Part 1

Questions

Section 1

Clinical methods and syndromes

1 Physical examination of a patient is facilitated by:

    a formulating a working diagnosis on the history
    b subdued lighting
    c a preliminary explanation of the purpose of the examination
    d excluding the accompanying relative or partner
    e background music

2 Heavy cigarette smoking is:

    a detected by inspecting the hands
    b associated with flushing and hyperventilation
    c produces shallow respiratory excursions
    d associated with a 'black hairy' tongue
    e associated with radiological changes in the lung

3 Examination of the hands commonly indicates the presence of:

    a acromegaly
    b chronic anaemia
    c diabetes mellitus
    d cyanotic heart disease
    e hyperthyroidism

4 Examination of the fingers facilitates the diagnosis of:

    a scleroderma
    b chronic lung disease
    c uraemia
    d rheumatoid arthritis
    e Cushing's syndrome

5 Examination of the tongue may reveal:

a candidiasis
b Crohn's disease
c Marfan's disease
d acromegaly
e Wilson's disease

6 A working diagnosis is:

a a clinical diagnosis arrived at by history and physical examination
b a diagnostic label that may change as new clinical data are assessed
c synonymous with the definitive diagnosis
d the diagnosis reached following elimination of all differential diagnoses
e the diagnosis used until clinical assessment is completed

7 Generalized oedema is associated with:

a renal failure
b haemochromatosis
c left heart failure
d snake bite
e chronic malnutrition

8 Water depletion clinically manifests as:

a anxiety and aggression
b muscle twitching
c oliguria
d tachycardia
e nausea and vomiting

9 Splenomegaly is a characteristic finding in:

a petechial haemorrhage
b disseminated intravascular coagulation
c hereditary telangiectasia
d von Willebrand's disease
e chronic malaria

10 A patient presenting with a bleeding diathesis may have:

  a undergone prosthetic heart valve surgery
  b suffered a snake bite
  c ingested a corrosive agent
  d a raised platelet count
  e had a mismatched blood transfusion

11 Chronic anaemia may present with:

  a exertional dyspnoea
  b hallucinations
  c a widened pulse pressure
  d hypopituitarism
  e diabetes insipidus

12 Anaemia due to defective erythropoiesis is an expected finding in the following diseases:

  a renal disease
  b iron deficiency states
  c hypersplenism
  d haemolytic–uraemic syndrome
  e hyperpituitarism

13 Chronic haemolytic anaemias commonly present with:

  a gallstones
  b splenomegaly
  c hepatomegaly
  d chronic leg ulceration
  e petechial haemorrhages

14 In a patient with a pyrexia of uncertain origin:

  a a definitive diagnosis is rarely made on the clinical findings
  b the diagnosis is usually of a rare disease
  c fever should have persisted for at least 30 days
  d a history of recent foreign travel is significant
  e the past medical history is usually not significant

15 **Chronic malnutrition is clinically associated with:**

    a anorexia nervosa
    b short bowel syndrome
    c bulimia nervosa
    d thyrotoxicosis
    e adhering to a high fibre, low fat diet

16 **An 18-year-old girl with Down's syndrome:**

    a is in control of her bodily functions
    b is amenorrhoeic
    c tends to be obese
    d has abnormalities of vision
    e is able to give a rudimentary history

17 **A 39-year-old man experienced facial sweating during eating on the side of recent parotid surgery. The condition is referred to as:**

    a Pierre Robin syndrome
    b Frey's syndrome
    c Sjögren–Larsen syndrome
    d Treacher Collins syndrome
    e Albright's syndrome

18 **Horner's syndrome is associated with:**

    a enophthalmos
    b benign apical lung disease
    c stroke (CVA)
    d loss of parasympathetic nerve supply to the eye
    e fifth cranial nerve palsy

19 **Crepitus on palpating a patient's chest is suggestive of:**

    a a keratotic skin lesion
    b subcutaneous emphysema
    c subcutaneous cellulitis
    d fractured rib(s)
    e a tumour undergoing central necrosis

20 Dysphagia:

    a is painful swallowing
    b may be associated with vomiting
    c is associated with oesophageal varices
    d may present with referred pain in the umbilicus
    e is a late feature of scleroderma

Section 2

Cutaneous lesions and infections

1 A keloid:

   a is poorly defined
   b has an irregular surface
   c may occur in any part of the body
   d is often seen following cosmetic surgery
   e is common over the sternum

2 Multiple subcutaneous nodules:

   a suggest an allergic phenomenon
   b may be neurofibromatosis
   c may be subcutaneous lipomata
   d are typically angiomas
   e are a feature of dermatomycosis

3 The features of cutaneous ulcer healing include:

   a the presence of granulation tissue
   b slough replacement by an eschar
   c an initial serious discharge becomes purulent
   d epithelialization
   e raising and eversion of the edges

4 A malignant ulcer is characterized by:

   a a 'punched out' base
   b rolled, everted edges
   c bleeding on contact
   d surrounding venous engorgement
   e an indurated base

5 A sinus:

  a is a tract lined with granulation tissue connecting two epithelial surfaces

  b is the end result of an unhealed ulcer

  c may result from malignant change in an ulcer

  d is a tract connecting an abnormal cavity to an epithelial surface

  e may result from poor healing in an implantation dermoid

6 Acute lymphangitis of the forearm presents with:

  a thrombosis of the superficial veins

  b ischaemic pain in the fingers

  c red streaking of the forearm

  d tender lymphadenopathy

  e swelling of the hand

7 A 37-year-old man presented with insidious ulceration of the scrotum. Examination revealed extensive necrosis of the scrotal skin and fascia. The diagnosis is:

  a a fulminating primary infection

  b a carcinoma

  c genital warts with secondary infection

  d lymphogranuloma venereum

  e a 'watering can' perineum

8 Inflammatory swelling and induration in the groin in an adult suggests a primary infective focus in the:

  a foot

  b abdominal wall

  c buttock

  d anus

  e perineum

9 An infection from a penetrating injury to the palm of the hand results in:

  a a subcutaneous inflammation and swelling

  b a mid-palmar space infection

  c an infection of the dorsal space

  d an infection of the tendon sheath

  e a claw hand

10 A tropical ulcer of the lower limb:

   a is always of infective origin
   b is usually pain-free and static
   c has a surrounding inflammatory reaction
   d with rolled, everted edges suggests malignant change
   e may produce a discharge of pigmented granules

11 Delayed wound healing is associated with:

   a local haematoma
   b jaundice
   c systemic steroid administration
   d primary suturing
   e an embedded foreign body

12 AIDS defining lesions in patients with seroconversion (AIDS-positive blood test) are:

   a Kaposi's sarcoma
   b hairy oral leukoplakia
   c cytomegalovirus retinitis
   d molluscum contagiosum
   e seborrhoeic dermatitis

13 Anal warts are:

   a diagnosed on inspection
   b associated with bleeding and pain
   c similar to penile warts
   d associated with procto-colitis
   e acquired through sexual contact

14 Clinical features following ingestion of a corrosive liquid are:

   a pupillary constriction
   b central chest pain radiating to the back
   c cardiac arrhythmia
   d pharyngeal oedema
   e coma due to toxic encephalitis

15 A sebacious horn is:

a caused by skin keratosis
b premalignant
c associated with skin tumours
d only found on the face
e characterized by ulceration and bleeding

**16 An adult presents with a 4-month history of a minimally
symptomatic red, raised, velvety plaque-like lesion involving the
corona and glans of an uncircumcised penis. The lesion is:**

a a penile wart
b Bowen's disease
c erythroplasia of Queyrat
d carcinoma-in-situ
e a rodent ulcer

17 A cutaneous malignant melanoma:

a is always pigmented
b is difficult to distinguish when arising from a pigmented
   mole
c presents with a generalized lymphadenopathy
d usually bleeds to touch
e may present with satellite lesions

18 A pilonidal sinus:

a occurs in the webs of fingers
b occurs in the umbilicus
c occurs in the natal cleft
d usually communicates with a visceral cavity
e rarely progresses to abscess formation

19 An umbilical erosion:

a is associated with a para-umbilical hernia
b is suggestive of intra-abdominal malignancy
c suggests a patent vitello-intestinal duct
d may result in a granuloma
e is rarely symptomatic

20 Acute appendicitis is:

a a clinical diagnosis
b associated with nausea, vomiting and generalized abdominal pain
c accompanied by tenesmus
d common in infancy
e difficult to diagnose in pregnancy

21 A pelvic abscess:

a points to the inner aspect of the thigh
b may cause diarrhoea
c is typically extraperitoneal
d collects in the Pouch of Douglas
e is detected by a gallium scan

Section 3

Injuries

1 Diagnostic features of shock in an injured patient include:

a hypotension and low cardiac output
b loss of consciousness
c central cyanosis
d inadequate perfusion of organs
e hypoxia and acidosis

2 Triage in trauma management is a system for:

a assessing injuries to establish treatment priorities
b sorting patients according to age
c selecting the most severely injured for priority treatment
d sorting the injured so that optimum use is made of available facilities
e allocating available medical personnel to patients with specific injuries

3 The primary survey of the multiply-injured patient is the:

a identification of treatable injuries
b identification of injuries requiring surgery
c identification of patients requiring immediate transfer to a specialist centre
d identification of life-threatening injuries and stabilizing the patient's condition
e correlation of injuries with causative factors and mechanisms

4 The secondary survey of the multiply-injured patient is:

a a method of identifying injuries missed in the primary survey
b taking a history and details of the injury-producing incident
c to identify and treat injuries not immediately life-threatening
d the assessment of all investigations requested in the primary survey
e the reassessment of injuries identified in the primary survey

5 A 19-year-old female gymnast fell off the parallel bars and complained of severe neck pain:

a passive neck movements may be gently elicited
b absence of cervical tenderness and muscle spasm excludes a cervical spinal injury
c a head injury may be safely excluded
d head and neck restraints may be removed if physical findings are negative
e cervical spine radiology should be requested as part of the primary survey

6 The following clinical findings in a patient suspected of internal injuries calls for urgent resuscitation:

a respiratory rate of 32 breaths/min
b temperature of 38.5°C
c pulse rate in excess of 120/min
d Glasgow Coma Scale of 8
e a distended abdomen

7 Following a crush injury to the chest:

a the main finding is an altered level of consciousness
b respiratory distress is usually associated with injury to the respiratory tract
c a pneumothorax is suggested by hyper-resonance and mediastinal shift
d paradoxical chest movements occur when adjacent ribs are fractured at one site
e a haemothorax is a rare complication

8 In a six-year-old child sustaining hot water scalds to the chest and abdomen, the:

a history of the incident is important
b area involved is approximately 18%
c injury is a partial thickness (second degree) burn
d child would be hypovolaemic
e child may return home following initial treatment

9 In a patient with a penetrating chest wound and cardiac tamponade there is:

a a raised CVP
b a high arterial pressure
c muffling of heart sounds
d a retrosternal pansystolic murmur
e a rise in CVP with inspiration

10 A 50% body surface burn in a conscious and orientated 70-year-old patient requires:

a adequate narcotic analgesia
b immediate resuscitation and life-support
c transfer to a major burns centre
d counselling on probable outcome
e seclusion with next of kin at bedside

11 A burn injury to an extremity:

a caused by electricity may produce ECG changes
b may produce laryngeal and pulmonary oedema
c that is full thickness produces little or no pain
d is limited to surface tissues
e is associated with emotional overlays

12 In a young adult with suspected smoke inhalation injury:

a the patient may be safely discharged home following a normal primary survey
b plain radiology of the chest will reveal any existing lung injury
c respiratory tract injury is likely
d ventilatory support in an intensive care setting may be required
e carbon monoxide poisoning may be excluded in the conscious patient

13 In a machine operator who sustained high tension electrical burns to his hand and buttock:

a the extent of the injury is usually confined to the entry and exit sites of the electric charge
b an immediate ECG is required
c the full extent of the injury will only become evident in the ensuing 72 hours
d renal failure is a likely complication
e ischaemic injury to the hand is a likely complication

14 In a cutaneous burn injury:

a the presence of blisters suggests a partial thickness (second degree) burn
b the presence of pain suggests a full thickness (third degree) burn
c a sero-sanguineous discharge indicates secondary infection
d significant tissue swelling is found only in a full thickness burn
e the colour of the exposed tissue is an indicator of burn depth

15 Frost bite of an extremity may be diagnosed by:

a hyperaemia and tissue swelling
b skin vesicle formation and blistering
c skin necrosis
d severe pain with skin blanching
e necrosis of muscle and bone

16 A pensioner was rescued from an unheated dwelling suffering from severe hypothermia and frostbite to both feet:

a the first priority is to attach a cardiac monitor and commence rewarming
b the surgical priority is to debride the frost-bitten tissues
c the initial line of demarcation is a good indicator of subsequent tissue survival
d the patient's insistence on returning home suggests cerebral hypoxia
e a flat ECG trace is a reliable indicator of death

17 In a 'blow-out' fracture of the orbit:

  a the floor of the orbit is usually intact
  b there is upward displacement of the eyeball
  c there is usually significant eye injury
  d double vision may be present
  e there is injury to the cutaneous innervation of the face

18 A cervical spine injury:

  a is not present if the patient has a normal range of
     painless active neck movements
  b may be safely detected by passive movement of the neck
  c is suggested by neck muscle spasm and pain
  d may be diagnosed by the mechanism of injury
  e is usually associated with injury to the head or upper
     thorax

**19 A 50-year-old lumberjack severed the sciatic nerve in the
    buttock in an accident involving a chain-saw; the clinical
    presentation is:**

  a foot drop
  b complete stocking anaesthesia
  c loss of knee flexion
  d loss of hip abduction
  e loss of active knee extension

20 In a tibial fracture:

  a the bone is not normally displaced if the fibula is intact
  b radiological delineation of the fracture site alone is
     sufficient
  c the presence of pedal pulses excludes a compartment
     syndrome
  d the mechanism of injury is unhelpful in assessing the
     injury and its complications
  e the fracture becomes a compound only when the fibula is
     also fractured

21 In a closed fracture of a long bone:

a absent distal pulses are due to vascular spasm
b the presence of crepitus suggests conversion to a compound fracture
c compartment syndrome is a potential complication
d there is minimal bleeding
e abnormal movements are absent

22 There is swelling, pain and bruising of the arm and elbow in an eight-year-old boy following a fall on his outstretched hand:

a he would hold his elbow in a flexed position
b dislocation of the elbow joint is possible
c a fracture of the lower end of the humerus is very unlikely
d passive extension of the elbow forms part of the examination
e sensation of the forearm and hand may be impaired

23 A 19-year-old man self-inflicted a laceration to his left wrist with division of the median nerve; the presentation is:

a wrist drop
b inability to oppose the thumb
c anaesthesia of the dorsum of the hand
d inability to abduct or adduct the fingers
e paralysis of finger flexion

24 In a man with a pelvic ring disruption injury sustained in a road traffic accident there was blood staining at the urethral meatus. The following are required to evaluate his injury:

a urethral catheterization
b urinalysis
c excretory urogram
d retrograde urethrogram
e CT scan of the pelvis

25 **Following the resolution of pain and swelling of an injured knee, a football player found the knee 'gave way' when weight bearing; the probable diagnosis is a:**

a   fracture of the articular surface
b   tear of the collateral ligament
c   tear of the cruciate ligament
d   tear of the patellar ligament
e   tear of the capsule

26 **A cricketer complains that his left knee suddenly locked whilst playing; he would:**

a   be unable to fully extend the knee
b   be unable to bend the knee
c   find the knee painful on weight bearing
d   find the knee fixed in a semi-flexed position
e   find the knee subluxed in the hyper-extended position

27 **A rugby player suffered severe pain and swelling over the anterior aspect of the knee on kicking a ball; he may present with the following:**

a   a locked knee
b   patellar dislocation
c   patellar fracture
d   knee joint dislocation
e   a torn medial meniscus

28 **The radiological findings that are suggestive of child abuse are:**

a   spiral fracture of the femur
b   growth plate injury
c   old scars from scalds or burns
d   multiple fractures in various stages of healing
e   a limb fracture with abundant new bone formation

29 **The signs of physical abuse in the elderly are:**

a   injuries to wrists and ankles
b   head injury
c   malnutrition and anaemia
d   multiple soft tissue contusions to face or body
e   anxiety with intension tremor

Head, face and neck

1 **Oral candidiasis was found in a 79-year-old woman admitted with an unrelated systemic illness; the diagnosis is suggested by the following:**

   a a black hairy tongue
   b red, raised plaques on the tongue
   c gingival ulcers
   d Koplik's spots on the oral mucosa
   e leukoplakia of the tongue

2 **A 59-year-old woman presents with an asymptomatic swelling in the right supra-clavicular fossa; the possible diagnoses are:**

   a a collar-stud abscess
   b subclavian artery aneurysm
   c a tumour deposit
   d an epidermoid cyst
   e a cervical rib

3 **A pulsatile lump on the side of the neck in a 83-year-old man would suggest the following:**

   a carotid body tumour
   b carotid aneurysm
   c mobile cervical lymph node
   d branchial cyst
   e lateral aberrant thyroid

4 **Acute raised intracranial pressure:**
   a is associated with headache and vomiting
   b leads to unconsciousness with dilated, sluggish pupil(s)
   c produces paralysis of the chorda tympani nerves
   d produces papilloedema
   e may lead to coning of the brain stem

5 **An epidural haemorrhage is distinguished from a subdural haemorrhage by a:**

   a fracture of the temporal bone overlying the middle meningeal artery
   b lucid interval
   c higher GCS score
   d sluggish pupillary reflex on the side of injury
   e contrast enhanced CT head scan

6 **An adult is admitted semi-conscious making incomprehensible noises and localizes painful stimuli; he is, however, unable to respond to verbal commands. He has a GCS score of:**

   a 4
   b 6
   c 8
   d 10
   e 12

7 **A young woman admitted as an emergency with a diagnosis of a subarachnoid haemorrhage would manifest the following:**

   a sudden and severe headache
   b dizziness and syncope
   c aphasia
   d third cranial nerve palsy
   e dysphagia

8 **A 56-year-old man developed a right-sided third cranial nerve palsy as a result of a Berry aneurysm of the right posterior communicating artery; he may present with:**

   a a right sided ptosis
   b a right dilated pupil
   c left external strabismus (squint)
   d double vision
   e blurring of left vision

9 Brain death in a comatose patient may be diagnosed:

a   in severe hypothermia with cardiac arrest
b   on a history of drug overdose
c   when cardio-respiratory function is dependent on ventilatory support
d   when clinical findings suggest a persistent vegetative state
e   in decorticate rigidity

10 In unilateral facial nerve injury there is:

a   loss of sensation over the cheek on the ipsilateral side
b   inability to wrinkle the forehead or grimace
c   facial asymmetry due to muscle action on the opposite side
d   difficulty with chewing
e   paralysis of the muscles of mastication

11 Carcinoma of the maxillary antrum in a 46-year-old wood worker typically presents with:

a   proptosis
b   toothache
c   swelling of the cheek
d   an ulcer on the hard palate
e   enlarged cervical lymph nodes

12 A patient with Bell's palsy has paralysis of the:

a   tongue
b   facial muscles
c   iris
d   sternomastoid muscle
e   stapedius

13 A four-year-old girl was found to have a hearing loss in one ear six months after an acute ear infection. A diagnosis of 'glue ear' was made and the clinical findings were:

a   a dry ear
b   ear pain
c   a bulging, inflamed ear drum
d   a perforated ear drum
e   behavioural problems

14 A patient with hearing loss:

a compensates by lip reading
b retains normal auditory acuity and speech discrimination if the loss is conductive
c may complain of auditory discomfort to high threshold sounds if there is cochlear damage
d rarely gives a history of exposure to unusually high noise levels
e is unlikely to give a relevant drug history

15 A patient suffering from vertigo:

a may exhibit symptoms of migraine or temporal lobe epilepsy
b experiences visual and auditory hallucinations
c experiences hallucinations of movement
d may have symptoms of Ménière's syndrome
e typically has conductive deafness

16 A painful red eye is characteristic of:

a keratitis
b bacterial conjunctivitis
c acute glaucoma
d scleritis
e anterior uveitis or iritis

17 A stone in the submandibular salivary gland duct presents with:

a a hard lump in the floor of the mouth
b purulent discharge in the floor of the mouth
c pain during chewing
d difficulty in swallowing
e a dry mouth

18 An 18-year-old man presents with an asymptomatic midline swelling in the front of his neck; the possible lesions are:

a a goitre
b a dermoid cyst
c a branchial cyst
d thymoma
e cystic hygroma

19 A thyroglossal cyst:

  a   presents as a lump on the back of the tongue
  b   is connected to the root of the tongue
  c   is stationary on swallowing
  d   moves when protruding the tongue
  e   may become infected and discharge into the mouth

20 A meningo-myelocoele in a neonate may present as:

  a   a swelling on the head
  b   a swelling over the back
  c   skin pigmentation or a tuft of hair
  d   paraplegia
  e   a midline posterior defect

Section 5

Endocrine and breast

1 In a patient presenting with Graves' disease the following serum parameters would be raised:

  a T4
  b thyrocalcitonin
  c total protein bound iodine (PBI)
  d thyroid stimulating antibodies
  e TSH

2 Thyrotoxicosis is characterized by:

  a weight loss
  b proximal myopathy
  c enophthalmos
  d tachycardia during sleep
  e nose bleeds

3 Myxoedema is characterized by:

  a fatigue
  b increased appetite
  c sweating
  d tremor
  e cardiac failure

4 Characteristic dermatological features of Cushing's syndrome include:

  a hypertrophy of the vascular elastic lamina
  b acne
  c plethoric facies
  d osteomalacia
  e hypertension

5 **A 29-year-old woman with biochemical evidence of anterior pituitary gland overactivity would present with:**
a telangiectatic skin lesions
b acne
c glycosuria
d Hippocratic facies
e buffalo hump

6 **In Addison's disease:**
a skin pigmentation occurs mainly in skin creases
b postural hypotension is characteristic
c anxiety and agitation are characteristic features
d there is fluid retention and peripheral oedema
e the patient may be admitted in hypovolaemic shock

7 **A goitre:**
a is any swelling arising in the front of the neck
b moves on swallowing
c is usually associated with hoarseness
d rarely produces thoracic inlet obstruction
e if painful is usually malignant

8 **Papillary carcinoma of the thyroid:**
a is associated with hoarseness
b is usually palpable
c spreads to cervical lymph nodes
d is associated with a bruit over the thyroid gland
e presents with bony metastases

9 **A 41-year-old woman with a medullary carcinoma of the thyroid gland may present with:**
a toxic symptoms
b ear ache
c hoarseness
d stridor
e enlarged cervical lymph nodes

10 A solitary nodule of the thyroid gland in a 32-year-old woman:

a is never malignant
b resolves with time
c requires radio-isotope scanning
d is a familial condition
e is not associated with toxicity

11 A 49-year-old man was diagnosed to have parathyroid overactivity; he would exhibit the following:

a hypercalcaemia
b tetany
c raised serum PO_4^- and lowered alkaline phosphatase
d labile hypertension
e personality changes

12 Parathyroid gland(s):

a overactivity is detected by Chvostek's sign
b are rarely palpable when hyperplastic or neoplastic
c are often mistaken for a lateral aberrant thyroid gland
d may be mistaken for enlarged cervical lymph nodes
e underactivity is detected by Trousseau's sign

13 Advanced breast cancer may present with:

a satellite lesions
b fibrocystic disease
c skin ulceration
d axillary lymphadenopathy
e inflammatory changes in the skin and subcutaneous tissue

14 A carcinoma of the breast in a 61-year-old woman is clinically staged as T_2 N_2 M_1; this implies:

a the tumour is more than 5 cm in size
b overlying skin is free of tumour
c axillary lymph nodes are palpable and mobile
d supraclavicular nodes are involved
e liver and/or bone involvement

15 An ulcerating lesion over a previously healthy mastectomy scar in a 63-year-old woman suggests:

a a benign ulcer of the chest wall
b a new cancer of the breast
c a recurrent cancer of the breast
d scar breakdown following chemotherapy
e scar breakdown following radiotherapy

16 Nipple discharge:

a is associated with pre-menstrual tension
b is a feature of Paget's disease
c is associated with duct ectasia
d if blood-stained may arise from fibrocystic disease
e if creamy is usually innocuous

17 The following types of nipple discharge in a 35-year-old woman are associated with:

a serous discharge with a duct papilloma
b milky discharge with lactation
c purulent discharge with Paget's disease of the nipple
d blood-stained discharge with duct ectasia
e greenish discharge with a ductal carcinoma

18 In a lactating 34-year-old woman presenting with pain, swelling and reddening of the right breast:

a the probable cause is breast engorgement
b the absence of a palpable lesion suggests acute mastitis
c the presence of a palpable lesion suggests an abscess
d the presence of palpable axillary nodes suggests an associated adenitis
e generalized breast inflammatory induration may suggest a carcinoma

19 A secretory focus that is situated away from the nipple–areolar complex of a lactating breast suggests:

a a mammary fistula
b a mammary sinus
c an accessory nipple
d duct ectasia
e a galactocoele

20 **A 30-year-old woman complaining of back pain, tiredness and paroxysmal headaches was found on isotope scanning to have a phaeochromocytoma. The clinical presentation includes:**

a   hypotension with syncope
b   labile hypertension
c   cardiac arrhythmias
d   a palpable tumour
e   renal failure

Section 6

Chest and spine

1 **A psoas abscess:**

   a often points in the groin
   b is associated with a vertebral lesion
   c is an extension of a perinephric abscess
   d presents as a fixed flexion deformity of the hip
   e presents as a sciatic nerve palsy

2 **Clinical indications of an inhalation injury are:**

   a history of a fire or explosion
   b facial scalds
   c singeing of the eyebrows and nasal vibrissae
   d carbonaceous sputum
   e history of impaired cerebration

3 **Carbon monoxide poisoning in a patient rescued from a fire is suggested by:**

   a history of exposure to fumes
   b headache and nausea
   c coma
   d hyperventilation and excitability
   e epileptic fits

4 **A pneumothorax in a 36-year-old woman is:**

   a rarely of the primary (spontaneous) variety
   b a complication of asthma
   c often associated with living at high altitude
   d commonly iatrogenic in origin
   e potentially fatal if of a tension variety

5 Empyema of the pleural cavity:

    a does not affect functional lung capacity
    b is characterized by dullness and reduced air entry on the affected side
    c increases vocal resonance on the affected side
    d rarely gives rise to purulent sputum
    e may progress to broncho-pleural fistula formation

6 Progressive respiratory failure is characterized by:

    a syncopic attacks
    b central cyanosis
    c pursing of lips during expiration
    d flaring of the ala nasi
    e venous congestion of the head and neck

7 Cough, haemoptysis and weight loss over a five-month period in a 65-year-old man suggest:

    a chronic respiratory infection
    b suppurative lung disease
    c bronchogenic carcinoma
    d chronic left ventricular failure
    e chronic obstructive airway disease

8 A 48-year-old cigarette smoker with a history of recurrent chest infections presented with a chronic cough and breathlessness. Bronchial carcinoma may be excluded if:

    a the chest infection has been ongoing or recurrent for a period exceeding two years
    b haemoptysis is not a feature
    c the cough is productive of copious purulent sputum
    d chest auscultatory findings are normal
    e there are no constitutional symptoms or loss of weight

9 A patient with an acute episode of angina pectoris exhibits:

    a central chest pain radiating down the right inner arm to the elbow and the little finger
    b severe chest pain radiating through to the back with circulatory collapse
    c breathlessness
    d nausea, profuse sweating and hypotension
    e hallucinations and dizziness leading to a faint

10 A 37-year-old woman with a diagnosis of aortic stenosis presents with:

a chest pain and syncopal attacks
b dyspnoea at rest
c a mid diastolic murmur, the duration of which indicates disease severity
d an ejection systolic murmur radiating to the carotids
e cor pulmonale

11 A 61-year-old man with stenosis of the mitral valve may present with:

a pulmonary hypertension
b ascites
c syncope
d splinter haemorrhages
e warm, flushed extremities

12 A neonate was found to cough and choke on feeds; chest auscultation revealed bilateral adventitious sounds. He may have:

a bronchopneumonia
b under-developed swallowing reflex
c oesophageal atresia
d a pharyngeal pouch
e tracheo-oesophageal fistula

13 Scoliosis of the spine is diagnosed by:

a a dorsal hump
b lateral angulation
c a gibbus deformity
d rotation of the rib cage
e measuring Cobb's angle

14 A 49-year-old man complains of chronic low backache that is progressive and exacerbated by physical activity. He may be suffering from:

a sciatica
b spinal stenosis
c ankylosing spondylitis
d osteoarthritis
e spondylolysthesis

15 In cervical spondylosis:

a presentation may be with severe headache
b all ages are affected
c symptoms may be referable to the upper limb
d physical activity exacerbates symptoms
e plain radiology of the neck is not usually diagnostic

16 A 17-year-old boy presents with a 10-week history of back pain. Examination revealed a dorsal spinal deformity and associated muscle spasm:

a fever and malaise suggest tuberculosis
b paraesthesia and lower limb weakness suggest spinal cord compression
c a fluctuant swelling over the spine suggests spinal caries
d hip muscle spasm suggests arthritis of that joint
e chronic cough with haemoptysis suggests tuberculosis

17 A 32-year-old woman with lateral prolapse of the C8–T1 intervertebral disc presents with:

a shoulder tip pain
b paraesthesia of the outer aspect of the upper arm
c weakness of the sternomastoid muscle
d weakness of the small muscles of the hand
e diminished or absent triceps jerk

18 A 36-year-old man with suspected spinal cord compression requires the following procedures for diagnostic confirmation:

a plain spinal radiology
b lumbar puncture
c MRI scan
d myelography
e spinal manometry

19 **A 65-year-old long-term male cigarette smoker presents with mild facial oedema, hoarseness, moderately distended neck veins, left sided Horner's syndrome and pain radiating down his left arm. These suggest:**

a   left recurrent laryngeal nerve palsy
b   superior vena caval obstruction
c   left sympathetic chain lesion
d   left brachial plexus lesion
e   nephrotic syndrome

20 **Injury to the long thoracic nerve of Bell presents as:**

a   inability to raise the arm above the head
b   inability to adduct the arm
c   loss of muscle power during pushing
d   loss of sensation to the upper six thoracic dermatomes
e   winging of the medial border of the scapula

Section 7

Abdomen

1 **A tender upper abdominal swelling in a 56-year-old woman with normal vital signs and a serum amylase of 900 IU suggests:**

   a acute phlegmonous pancreatitis
   b haemorrhagic pancreatitis
   c pseudocyst of the pancreas
   d pancreatic abscess
   e pancreatic tumour

2 **In an eight-year-old Asian child with massive hepatosplenomegaly the causative disease states are:**

   a malaria
   b visceral leishmaniasis
   c sickle cell disease
   d coeliac disease
   e Budd–Chiari syndrome

3 **In acute necrotizing pancreatitis:**

   a there is a palpable upper abdominal mass
   b the signs are identical to those of generalized peritonitis
   c hypovolaemic shock is likely
   d serum amylase level may not reflect the severity of the disease
   e serum calcium is raised

4 **Abdominal aortic aneurysms:**

   a frequently dissect
   b are usually asymptomatic
   c may be diagnosed on plain abdominal radiography
   d have an increased incidence in diabetics
   e may produce acute lower limb ischaemia

5 The physical findings that assist in the diagnosis of inguinal herniae are:

a   a direct hernia lies above and medial to the pubic tubercle

b   the hernia in relation to the pulsation of the inferior epigastric artery determines its type

c   a direct hernia produces a negative cough impulse following reduction and occlusion of the internal ring

d   occlusion of the external ring produces a negative cough impulse from an indirect hernia

e   an indirect hernia lies below and lateral to the pubic tubercle

6 An umbilical hernia is:

a   commoner in babies than in adolescents

b   associated with umbilical ring piercing

c   prone to strangulation

d   not usually associated with a cough impulse

e   associated with ascites

7 Hepatomegaly is:

a   the clinical presentation of a hepatoma

b   associated with anaemia

c   usually accompanied by jaundice

d   associated with portal hypertension

e   associated with fluid retention

8 A 73-year-old woman with a pancreatic cancer may present with:

a   jaundice

b   a non-tender upper abdominal mass

c   diabetes mellitus

d   thrombophlebitis migrans

e   pancreatic calcinosis

9 A patient with Peutz–Jeghers syndrome may:

a   show failure to thrive

b   present with melaena

c   have pigmentation of the lips

d   have bowel polyps

e   present with bowel obstruction

10 Common presentations of Crohn's disease include:

a dyspepsia and heart burn
b fever and crampy abdominal pain
c tenesmus with fresh rectal bleeding
d sub-acute bowel obstruction
e bloody diarrhoea and an abdominal mass

11 Causes of severe rectal bleeding are:

a diverticular disease
b angiodysplasia
c ischaemic colitis
d haemorrhoids
e colonic carcinoma

12 A 33-year-old stock-market trader complains of severe upper abdominal pain relieved by eating with a marked periodicity over a nine-month period; other probable symptoms are:

a dyspepsia and flatulence
b heartburn
c halitosis
d loss of appetite
e nocturnal pain

13 A 34-year-old doctor returning from working in a refugee camp in Eastern Europe develops features suggestive of an acute liver abscess; these are:

a swinging pyrexia
b jaundice
c tender hepatomegaly
d pleural effusion
e leucocytosis

14 A 26-year-old woman was referred with a suspected diagnosis of acute appendicitis; the positive findings are:

a foetor oris
b tenesmus
c guarding and rigidity in the right lower abdominal quadrant
d hyperactive bowel sounds
e tenderness on pelvic examination

15 Small bowel obstruction:

a presents with abdominal pain and vomiting
b is preceded by constipation
c has a diagnostic radiological ladder pattern
d may present as gallstone ileus
e may present as a silent abdomen

16 A 28-year-old male AIDS sufferer presents with non-specific abdominal symptoms and is found to have a colonic intussusception on CT scanning; the clinical findings are:

a abdominal guarding and rigidity
b hypovolaemia
c pyrexia and toxaemia
d hyperactive bowel sounds
e a normal rectal examination

17 A neonate presents with projectile vomiting following feeds and his mother noticed a transient firm lump in his abdomen soon after. The probable diagnoses are:

a achalasia of the cardia
b hiatus hernia
c volvulus of the stomach
d hypertrophic pyloric stenosis
e duodenal atresia

18 An infant with congenital megacolon presents with:

a abdominal distension
b constipation alternating with diarrhoea
c increased bowel sounds
d meconium ileus
e a distended rectum

19 A 79-year-old man with an adenocarcinoma (hypernephroma) of the kidney may present with:

a clot colic
b febrile episodes
c a pathological fracture
d a rapidly developing varicocoele
e polycythaemia

20 Renal colic is:

a associated with nausea and loin tenderness
b referred to the testis
c usually due to calculus
d accompanied by haematuria
e usually accompanied by renal damage

Section 8

Pelvis

1 Transillumination is positive in the following scrotal lesions:

   a lipoma
   b varicocoele
   c vaginal hydrocoele
   d haematocoele
   e spermatocoele

2 An indirect inguinal hernia:

   a is caused by a defect in the posterior wall of the inguinal canal
   b arises lateral to the inferior epigastric artery
   c passes below and medial to the pubic tubercle
   d may strangulate
   e may present as a large scrotal swelling

3 A femoral hernia:

   a is more common in the obese
   b is often bilateral
   c may present with a cough impulse in the groin
   d lies above and medial to the pubic tubercle
   e may lie in the upper part of the scrotum

4 A patient with early carcinoma of the rectum may present with:

   a tenesmus and a sense of incomplete emptying
   b spurious diarrhoea with loss of continence
   c nausea and loss of appetite
   d severe anaemia and cachexia
   e mucosal prolapse

5 Haemorrhoids:

a are the commonest cause of bleeding following defecation
b usually present with pain
c are associated with low intrasphincteric pressures
d are associated with constipation
e may regress to form anal skin tags

6 Rectal prolapse:

a may present with tenesmus and bleeding
b is commonly found in the very young and the elderly
c involving mucosal prolapse is distinguished from full thickness prolapse by palpation
d is associated with ulcerative colitis
e may predispose to ulceration and gangrene

7 A 59-year-old man with prostatic symptoms is diagnosed on digital rectal examination to have a prostatic cancer; the positive findings include a:

a tender enlarged prostate
b firm nodular prostate
c tethering of the rectal wall
d firm normal-sized prostate
e hard, craggy prostate

8 Chronic urinary retention is:

a due to urethral calculus obstruction
b associated with suprapubic pain and tenderness
c associated with a constant desire to void
d associated with a palpable urinary bladder
e usually accompanied by upper tract dilatation

9 The urinary bladder is:

a rarely palpable in chronic urinary retention
b usually palpable when it contains a large vesical calculus
c usually palpable when containing a tumour
d readily identifiable on plain radiology when distended
e liable to rupture when acutely distended

10 **A 62-year-old woman under surveillance for transitional cell carcinoma of the bladder, treated by cystoscopic resection, develops symptoms suggestive of a recurrence; they include:**

a   perineal pain or discomfort
b   painless haematuria
c   clot retention
d   strangury
e   bladder outflow obstruction

11 **A nine-year-old Asian boy was found to have a vesical stone on plain abdominal radiology. His clinical presentation would include:**

a   frequency of micturition
b   pain referred to the tip of the penis at the end of micturition
c   haematuria at the end of micturition
d   strangury
e   pyuria

12 **A 37-year-old woman with a clinical diagnosis of chronic pyelonephritis is likely to present with:**

a   a dull ache in the loin
b   a normal blood pressure
c   a normochromic, normocytic anaemia
d   casts in the urine
e   a high urinary white cell count

13 **A 27-year-old man is diagnosed to have chronic prostatitis; the clinical presentation is:**

a   fever with rigors
b   pain on micturition
c   prostatic tenderness on rectal examination
d   threads in the urine
e   pelvic pain following sexual intercourse

14 An inflammatory urethral stricture in a 29-year-old man presents with:

a straining to void
b dribbling
c acute urinary retention
d a morning 'dew drop'
e a periurethral abscess

15 A painful chronic genital ulcer is:

a caused by herpes
b caused by syphilis
c usually associated with pelvic and/or para-aortic lymphadenopathy
d usually accompanied by groin lymphadenopathy
e associated with recurrent discharge

16 A 21-year-old man presented with a six-month history of testicular symptoms; a clinical diagnosis of a testicular tumour was made on the following:

a a painless swelling of the scrotum
b a right hypochondrial mass
c para-aortic nodal enlargement
d haemospermia
e azoospermia

17 A vaginal hydrocoele is:

a transilluminant
b distinct from an epididymal cyst on palpation
c associated with a scrotal hernia
d associated with a cystocoele of the vagina
e associated with a 'watering can' perineum

18 Testicular torsion in a 15-year-old boy:

a must be confirmed by ultrasound scan
b presents with dysuria
c must be treated within four hours of onset of symptoms
d predisposes to torsion of the contralateral testis
e is associated with a vaginal hydrocoele

19 Iliac vein thrombosis in a previously healthy 36-year-old-woman:

a   presents with pelvic discomfort and/or backache
b   is usually accompanied by deep tenderness on pelvic examination
c   is usually devoid of physical signs
d   is potentially life-threatening
e   cannot be diagnosed by vascular imaging

20 In a male neonate with complete ectopia vesicae, the clinical features are:

a   a defect in the abdominal wall
b   epispadias
c   visible ureteric orifices
d   an associated para-umbilical hernia
e   absence of an umbilicus

Section 9

Limbs

1 An inability to extend the fingers is caused by:

    a carpal tunnel syndrome
    b Volkmann's ischaemic contracture
    c Dupuytren's contracture
    d full thickness burn injury to the dorsum of the hand
    e an upper motor neurone lesion

2 A seven-year-old girl with stunted growth and bowing of the legs:

    a has osteomalacia
    b probably has rickets
    c is malnourished
    d has little need for radiology for a diagnosis
    e may have a greenstick fracture of the leg

3 Diabetic ulcers of the foot:

    a are due to vascular disease
    b are due to neuropathic skin changes
    c may result in haemorrhage
    d may extend to involve the joints
    e eventually leads to malignant change

4 The clinical findings in a patient presenting with an ingrowing toe-nail are:

    a ischaemic changes to the toe
    b bleeding from the nail-bed
    c swelling and tenderness of the nail bed
    d ulceration with discharge from the nail fold
    e pain and stiffness of the interphalangeal joint

5 Dry gangrene of an extremity is characterized by:

a oedema and mottling
b skin discoloration with demarcation
c painless skin changes
d anaerobic tissue metabolism
e crepitus on palpation

6 Intermittent claudication:

a comes on at rest
b is characterized by 'venous guttering'
c improves after coronary artery by-pass surgery
d is improved by regular exercise
e may precede critical limb ischaemia

7 Ischaemic foot ulceration:

a occurs mainly on heels and toes
b is associated with normal arterial limb pulses
c is associated with venous bleeding
d may be painless in diabetes
e is associated with a low ankle pressure index

8 Raynaud's phenomenon of the hands is:

a accentuated in liver disease
b caused by vasospasm
c characterized by digital redness on exposure to cold
d associated with the use of vibrating tools
e commonly found in young women

9 Varicose veins of the lower limb:

a are obvious on inspection
b may show trophic changes in the overlying skin
c are pulsatile when communicating with deep veins
d disappear on raising the leg
e predispose to ulceration

10 Lymphoedema of the lower limb:

a may present with weakness and paraesthesia
b may present with stiffness and swelling
c is associated with venous insufficiency
d predisposes to infection
e predisposes to phlegmasia alba dolens (white leg)

11 A 36-year-old woman complains of progressive pain and
    stiffness in her lower back, with pain radiating down the right
    buttock and thigh over a four-month period; more recently she
    experienced pins and needles sensation in the calf and foot.
    These symptoms are characteristic of:

    a   disc degeneration or prolapse
    b   multiple sclerosis
    c   spinal canal tumour
    d   TB of the lumbar spine
    e   idiopathic scoliosis

12 A febrile nine-year-old boy gives a two-week history of pain
    and swelling in the region of his left knee:

    a   fluctuation may be elicited
    b   septic arthritis is a likely diagnosis
    c   osteomyelitis is a likely diagnosis
    d   he classically has a pathological fracture
    e   diagnosis is made by plain radiology of the joint

13 In Paget's disease of the tibia:

    a   the patient is usually symptomatic
    b   there is bone sclerosis with thickening
    c   the bone is brittle
    d   the deformity is called 'sabre tibia'
    e   all ages are affected

14 A patient with a primary tumour of the femur may present
    with:

    a   a tender swelling in the thigh
    b   a pathological fracture
    c   plain radiology showing 'sun ray' spicules
    d   plain radiology showing 'soap bubble' appearance
    e   foot drop

15 The clinical features of rheumatoid arthritis are:

    a   weakness and loss of appetite
    b   joint ankylosis
    c   tenosinovitis
    d   deformity of affected joints
    e   sclerosis of bones of affected joints

16 A positive Trendelenburg test:

a produces a lurching gait downwards on the unsupported side
b on both sides results in an apparently normal gait
c is when the pelvis rises on the unsupported side on walking
d is detected by measuring limb length
e is found following non-union of a femoral neck fracture

17 In a patient complaining of pain and stiffness of the hip, the following observations assist in making a diagnosis:

a limb deformity
b limb measurements
c passive range of movements
d gait
e limb sensation

18 A mother complained that her six-month-old infant has a lop-sided crawl and the legs do not open properly for nappy changes. An abnormal fold of skin is noticed over the thigh with apparent shortening of that limb. A diagnosis may be reached by:

a genetic testing for chromosomal abnormalities
b Ortolani's test
c Barlow's test
d ultra-sound scan of the hip joints
e neurological assessment of the limbs

19 A healthy 10-year-old school girl complains of progressive pain in her hip and a limp for five months, she:

a may have a palpable swelling of the hip joint
b may have Perthes' disease
c may have a slipped femoral epiphysis
d is likely to have a lesion in the lumbosacral spine
e is likely to have a full range of hip movements

20 The clinical features associated with the diagnosis of a chronic slipped upper femoral epiphysis are:

a   a positive Trendelenburg test
b   lengthening of the limb
c   restricted external rotation and adduction
d   pain referred to the knee
e   fixed flexion deformity of the hip

21 The clinical findings of osteoarthritis of the hip are:

a   nocturnal pain that wakes the patient
b   wasting of the glutei
c   progressive restriction of movement
d   limb lengthening
e   telescopic movement

22 In osteoarthritis of the knee:

a   there is pain and stiffness
b   there is no joint deformity
c   extension may be restricted
d   the joint occasionally 'locks'
e   plain radiology is diagnostic

23 A 59-year-old woman with a total hip replacement three years previously, complains of pain in the groin radiating to the thigh resulting in a progressive limp. Diagnosis includes:

a   chronic low grade infection in the joint
b   loosening of the prosthesis
c   periprosthetic fracture
d   acute dislocation
e   heterotropic bone formation

24 The clinical findings in an adolescent with club foot are:

a   adduction of the forefoot
b   wasting of calf muscles
c   abnormality of the calcaneum (os calcis)
d   limb shortening
e   the toes are vestigial or absent

Part 2

Answers and comments

Clinical methods and syndromes

1 Physical examination of a patient is facilitated by:

a – true, b – false, c – true, d – false, e – false

It is usual to arrive at a working diagnosis following a good history in over 80% of patients, physical examination and investigations serving only to confirm. The clinician should conduct the interview in an atmosphere that avoids stress and enhances patient confidence. Lighting must be optimum to demonstrate signs; extraneous noises, e.g. piped music, serve only to distract. When relatives wish to be present at the examination, their numbers should be limited to one or two who are closely involved as parents, guardians or carers.

Ch 1, p. 2–5

2 Heavy cigarette smoking is:

a – true, b – true, c – false, d – true, e – true

It is important to identify heavy smoking in patients who require major surgery in time to improve their respiratory reserves. Broncho-vascular lung markings are typically more marked on plain radiology in smokers; smoking compromises tissue vascularity and delays healing. Stopping smoking is a pre-requisite for transplant and prosthetic surgery and for vascular reconstruction.

Ch 1, p. 6, *Fig 1.5*
Ch 28, p. 363
Fig 13.36

3 Examination of the hands commonly indicates the presence of:

a – true, b – true, c – false, d – true, e – true

The hands portray the health and the way of life of the subject; they often reveal stigmata of systemic disease. Note the strength of the grip, the warmth and dryness of the skin when shaking hands. Finger joints may exhibit bony thickenings, e.g. Heberden's nodules at the base of the terminal phalanges in osteoarthritis and spindle-shaped swellings of the interphalangeal joints in rheumatoid arthritis. Trophic skin changes may be present in neurological and peripheral vascular diseases. Tremor may be familial or due to nervousness, senility or alcoholism; of greater significance are tremors of liver and/or renal failure, or those caused by neurological (e.g. multiple sclerosis, Parkinsonism) and endocrine (e.g. thyrotoxicosis, acromegaly) disease. Wasting of the small muscles of the hand and deformities of the hand are produced by peripheral nerve lesions and fascial contractures (Dupuytren's, burns scarring).

Ch 1, p. 6–10, *Fig 1.1, 1.2, 1.3, 1.4, 1.5, 1.17, 1.29, 1.30, 1.31, 1.32, 1.33*

4 Examination of the fingers facilitates the diagnosis of:

a – true, b – true, c – false, d – true, e – false

Nail abnormalities such as brittleness, discoloration and clubbing suggest nutritional, haematological, pulmonary or cardiac disease states. In subacute bacterial endocarditis in addition to clubbing, painful nodules at the fingertips (Osler's nodes) and 'splinter haemorrhages' in nail beds are characteristic. Nail bed infarcts are seen in micro-thromboemboli, polyarteritis and systemic lupus erythematosus.

Ch 1, p. 6–10, *Fig 1.6, 1.7, 1.8, 1.9, 1.10, 1.11, 1.12, 1.13, 1.14, 1.16*

5   Examination of the tongue may reveal:

a – true, b – true, c – false, d – true, e – false

When requesting the patient to protrude the tongue, the inability to do so fully may be due to tongue-tie, palsy or carcinomas of the tongue or the floor of the mouth. Tissue hydration is assessed by the surface moisture and anaemia or central cyanosis by its colour. A large tongue may suggest acromegaly, cretinism, myxoedema or amyloidosis. Tremor may be due to nervousness, thyrotoxicosis or Parkinsonism. Hypoglossal nerve lesion produces hemiatrophy and deviation. Loss of surface papillae denotes vitamin B12 or iron deficiency (pellagra); it is also seen in some malabsorption syndromes (coeliac disease). A dry brown tongue is a late stage of some severe illnesses.

Ch 1, p. 12–14, *Fig 1.45, 1.47, 1.48, 1.49*
Ch 13, p. 196–8, *Fig 13.35, 13.36, 13.37, 13.38*

6   A working diagnosis is:

a – true, b – true, c – false, d – false, e – true

The concept of a working diagnosis arises from the problem orientated medical recording system of entering and updating clinical and laboratory data on patients. It is based on the evolving nature of the diagnosis and does away with a list of differential diagnoses that require elimination. The working diagnosis is made during the first clinical contact with the patient and revised on the results of ongoing investigations which incorporates disease progression, complications, remission and relapses.

Ch 1, p. 15

7 Generalized oedema is associated with:

a – true, b – false, c – false, d – true, e – true

Generalized oedema is caused either by fluid retention or by an acute inflammatory reaction. Acute generalized body swelling is usually only seen as a manifestation of severe allergic reaction (anaphylaxis). This is usually triggered by the ingestion or inoculation of a foreign protein. In addition to food allergies, drugs, insect bites and vaccines are occasional causes. Angioedema causes diffuse swelling of loose connective tissue of mucous membranes of the eyelids, lips and genitalia. Glottic oedema produces respiratory distress and the accompanying stridor and should not be mistaken for an asthmatic attack.

Ch 2, p. 19–21, *Fig 2.1*
Fig 1.34

8 Water depletion clinically manifests as:

a – false, b – true, c – true, d – true, e – false

Water depletion is shared by the intracellular and extracellular fluid spaces and affects transcellular ion exchange and cellular metabolism. The clinical signs are generally non-specific and changes in mental state are usually the most obvious; they vary from subtle changes in personality to irritability, hyper-reflexia, seizures and coma. When mild, the only signs are diminished skin turgor and reduced intraocular tension. When the extracellular volume diminishes by 5% or more orthostatic tachycardia and/or hypotension with decreased CVP are detectable. Serum urea and electrolyte and urine output give an accurate estimation of fluid and electrolyte loss for replacement therapy.

Ch 2, p. 22–3

9 Splenomegaly is a characteristic finding in:

a – true, b – false, c – false, d – false, e – true

Abnormalities of the spleen are almost always due to primary disorders elsewhere. Lymphoproliferative, myeloproliferative and connective tissue diseases along with chronic parasitic infestations (e.g. malaria, kala-azar) lead to splenic enlargement. Hypersplenism which is associated with blood dyscrasias also produces spenomegaly leading to a reduction in one or more blood cell elements resulting in anaemia, leukopenia and/or thrombocytopenia with hyperplasia of bone marrow cell precursors.

Ch 2, p. 23–5, *Fig 2.11*

10 A patient presenting with a bleeding diathesis may have:

a – true, b – true, c – false, d – false, e – false

Bleeding diatheses are produced by a deficiency of one or more coagulation factors or can be due to disseminated intravascular coagulation. Major bleeding occurs in 3–5% of patients on long-term anticoagulant therapy and details of the latter must be obtained. Purpuric patches and spontaneous bruising may be clinically apparent and evidence of occult bleeding is obtained from examining the urine and the stool.

Ch 2, p. 25–7, *Fig 2.14*

11 Chronic anaemia may present with:

a – true, b – false, c – true, d – true, e – false

The clinical manifestations of anaemia are related to its severity and duration, as they are caused by tissue hypoxia with compensatory respiratory and vascular responses. Symptoms of severe anaemia are weakness, vertigo, headache, tinnitus, spots before the eyes, easy fatiguability, drowsiness, irritability and psychological aberrations. Amenorrhoea, loss of libido, low grade fever, gastrointestinal upsets and congestive heart failure may also occasionally develop.

Ch 2, p. 27–32

12 Anaemia due to defective erythropoiesis is an expected finding in the following diseases:

a – true, b – true, c – false, d – false, e – false

Defective erythropoiesis is due to bone marrow failure or to deficiency of erythropoietic factors such as iron, copper, cobalt, vitamin B12 and folic acid. Hypoplastic and aplastic anaemias may be idiopathic or familial (Fanconi syndrome). Exposure to industrial chemicals (e.g. benzene, arsenic), irradiation or cancer chemotherapy may result in aplastic anaemia. Waxy skin and mucous membrane pallor is characteristic. Thrombocytopenia may produce bleeding into these structures and leukopenia may result in respiratory infections.

Ch 2, p. 27–9, *Fig 2.15, 2.16*

13 Chronic haemolytic anaemias commonly present with:

a – true, b – true, c – false, d – true, e – false

Haemolytic anaemia occurs when the red cell life span is foreshortened and not compensated by accelerated red cell production. Haemolysis generally occurs extravascularly and the resulting splenic enlargement and hypersplenism jeopardize normal red cell survival. Intravascular haemolysis results in haemoglobinuria and jaundice is a feature of both. Haemolysis may be acute, chronic or episodic. Acute, severe haemolysis (haemolytic crisis, e.g. in sickle cell disease) is uncommon and is accompanied by chills, fever and abdominal, back or limb pains leading to prostration and shock. Jaundice occurs when the liver's capacity to convert haemoglobin to conjugated bilirubin is overwhelmed and unconjugated bilirubin spills over into the circulation.

Ch 2, p. 31
Fig 29.25(g)

14 In a patient with a pyrexia of uncertain origin:

a – true, b – false, c – false, d – true, e – false

Pyrexia of uncertain origin is a body temperature of 38.5°C
or higher on four or more occasions over a period of two weeks.
In adults, TB, occult infections of the kidney, brain, liver or
peritoneal cavity are likely causes. Collagen diseases,
inflammatory bowel disease, subacute bacterial endocarditis and
blood and lymphatic cancers are other causes. In children
infections (viral and bacterial) are presumed to cause the vast
majority of such fevers; upper respiratory viral infections are
prominent under two years of age whilst infectious
mononucleosis and endocarditis should be considered over the
age of six.

Ch 2, p. 33

15 Chronic malnutrition is clinically associated with:

a – true, b – false, c – false, d – true, e – false

Mild to moderate protein–calorie-malnutrition is best assessed by
anthropometry; it is estimated by calculating weight as a
percentage of expected weight/height/(age in children), normal
being 90–110%, mild 85–90%, moderate 75–85%, and severe
< 75%. In children there is growth retardation in addition to the
effects of marasmus or kwashiorkor in severe cases. The latter is
characterized by oedema, 'flaky paint' dermatosis, thinning and
decoloration of the hair, enlarged fatty liver and apathy.

Ch 2, p. 34–5

16 An 18-year-old girl with Down's syndrome:

a – false, b – false, c – true, d – true, e – false

Intellectual and motor functions are severely impaired in Down's
syndrome; facial characteristics are readily recognized but the
presence of a simian palmar crease is variable. Affected children
and adolescents are usually oblivious to most ailments and the
history is obtained from their carers and examination requires
their participation in soothing and comforting the patient.

Ch 2, p. 42, *Fig 2.42, 2.43*

17 A 39-year-old man experienced facial sweating during eating on the side of recent parotid surgery. The condition is referred to as:

a – false, b – true, c – false, d – false, e – false

Frey's syndrome results in the abnormal re-innervation of the cervical sympathetic fibres following traumatic injury. Developmental abnormalities of the facial bones give rise to Pierre Robin and Treacher Collins syndromes. In Albright's syndrome cystic bone lesions may present with endocrine abnormalities and skin pigmentation.

Ch 9, p. 160

18 Horner's syndrome is associated with:

a – true, b – true, c – false, d – false, e – false

Horner's syndrome is the result of the loss of the sympathetic innervation to the eye. This may be due to lesions arising in the brain stem, cervical cord or the sympathetic chain. They may be caused by trauma; ischaemic changes; degenerative changes, e.g. syringobulbia, syringomyelia; and compression or invasion of the cervical nerve roots, e.g. apical lung infection (TB) and Pancoast tumour. The result is a sunken eye with pupillary constriction, ptosis and loss of sweating on the ipsilateral side of the face.

Ch 12, p. 185, *Fig 12.52*
Fig 31.2

19 Crepitus on palpating a patient's chest is suggestive of:

a – false, b – true, c – false, d – true, e – false

Crepitus is the sign, sine qua non, elicited by the palpating hand, indicating the presence of subcutaneous gas. The grating sensation felt when moving an arthritic joint or when ends of a broken bone grate against each is also referred to as crepitus.

Ch 19, p. 241, *Fig 19.1*
Ch 38, p. 474, *Fig 38.4*

20 Dysphagia:

a – false, b – true, c – false, d – false, e – true

Dysphagia is difficulty in swallowing; a working diagnosis is usually arrived at on the history as the oesophagus is inaccessible to clinical examination. The cause is usually a stricture (inflammatory or neoplastic) or due to muscular incoordination. The history is usually of gradual onset of symptoms with progression. Inflammatory strictures are a sequela to ingestion of corrosives whilst malignant strictures, though insidious in onset, are rapidly progressive and lead to weight loss and inanition. Functional causes include motor neurone disease where the symptoms are progressive. Oesophagoscopy and biopsy identify mural lesions whilst manometry reveals abnormalities in neuromuscular conduction.

Ch 19, p. 250–2, *Fig 19.29, 19.31*

Section 2

Cutaneous lesions and infections

1 A keloid:

a – false, b – true, c – true, d – false, e – true

A scar is the result of healing following injury or destruction of the skin layers. Surgical scars are easily recognized and inspection provides the following information:

- the surrounding erythema or pallor indicates whether the operation was recent or not;
- the anatomic site and scar length suggests the type of surgery and its magnitude;
- hypertrophic scarring suggests delayed healing due to tissue malnutrition or sepsis;
- the positioning, the contour and the regularity of the scar may indicate whether cosmetic factors were taken into account during surgery.

Ch 3, p. 48–50, *Fig 3.5*
Ch 4, p. 81–2, *Fig 4.63, 4.64, 4.65*
Ch 8, p. 137, *Fig 8.28*

2 Multiple subcutaneous nodules:

a – false, b – true, c – true, d – false, e – false

When palpating a subcutaneous lump in order to deduce its nature, the 'slipping sign' of a lipoma is elicited when it moves away from the examining finger; a cystic swelling may be shown to fluctuate in two planes; a fibroma is firm in texture and, due to its fibrous tetherings, less mobile. Multiple fatty or fibro-fatty lumps may occasionally be painful or tender to palpation, particularly when located over 'pressure areas'; there is usually a family history of such lesions.

Ch 3, p. 48–52, *Fig 3.14*

3   The features of cutaneous ulcer healing include:

a – true, b – true, c – false, d – true, e – false

Skin ulcers are the result of loss of the epidermis and part or all
of the dermis. The commonest cause of poor healing is infection
and/or malnutrition. Chronic infections, peripheral vascular
disease, cutaneous neuropathies, autoimmune disease and cancers
also produce ulcers and diagnosis requires identification of the
underlying disease. Self-inflicted ulcers are rare, and difficult to
diagnose and treat.

Ch 3, p. 56–7, *Fig 3.28*

4   A malignant ulcer is characterized by:

a – false, b – true, c – true, d – false, e – true

Malignant ulceration of an epithelial surface is often the result
of pre-existing changes brought on by chronic irritation from
physical or chemical agents. The following changes in a
pre-existing lesion suggest a malignant ulcer: ulceration in a
mole or in an area of actinic keratosis; recent change in a benign
ulcer; and rapid extension.

Ch 3, p. 55–8, *Fig 3.36*

5   A sinus:

a – false, b – false, c – true, d – true, e – true

A sinus is a tract that connects an epithelial surface with a cavity
lined with granulation tissue. This usually results in a chronic
discharging focus which persists until the inflammatory process in
the cavity resolves. A discharging sinus is usually the culmination
of an unresolved focus of infection and is found typically in
branchial and thyroglossal sinuses in the neck and pilonidal
sinuses in the webs of fingers, the umbilicus and the natal cleft.

Ch 3, p. 58–9, *Fig 3.37, 3.38*

6 Acute lymphangitis of the forearm presents with:

a – false, b – false, c – true, d – true, e – true

Lymphangitis is inflammation of the regional lymphatic channels as a result of sepsis arising in the area of drainage. The lymph nodes draining the area become inflamed and palpable. The site of entry of the infection, the primary focus of infection, is usually a pulp or a nail bed infection and must be identified.

Ch 4, p. 63, *Fig 4.2*
Ch 29, p. 393, *Fig 29.25(o)*

7 A 37-year-old man presented with insidious ulceration of the scrotum. Examination revealed extensive necrosis of the scrotal skin and fascia. The diagnosis is:

a – true, b – false, c – false, d – false, e – false

Fournier's gangrene (of the scrotum) is a primary mixed bacterial infection. Predisposing factors are chronic malnutrition, diabetes and perianal sepsis. Inflammatory oedema of the scrotum leads to rapid sloughing of the tissues due to compromised viability with the exposure of the testes and cord structures. Progression of the infection to scrotal contents results in thrombosis of the testicular vessels and gangrene.

Ch 4, p. 64
Ch 27, p. 356–7, *Fig 27.34, 27.35*

8 Inflammatory swelling and induration in the groin in an adult suggests a primary infective focus in the:

a – true, b – true, c – true, d – true, e – true

A tender, indurated swelling(s) of the groin with or without systemic symptoms may represent either an incarcerated groin hernia or inflammation of the inguinal lymph nodes. These are the watershed to the lymphatics draining the lower limb, perineum, buttock and the lower abdominal wall on that side. Primary tumours in these regions may present with metastatic deposits in the groin or along the lymphatics draining the tumour. Squamous carcinoma of the anus may metastasize to the inguinal as well as to the aorto-iliac nodes.

Ch 4, p. 64–6, *Fig 4.5*

9   An infection from a penetrating injury to the palm of the hand results in:

a – false, b – true, c – false, d – true, e – true

This infection is caused by a penetrating wound entering a flexor tendon sheath in the palm leading to a fulminating infection in the confined space producing swelling and severe pain. Active or passive flexion of the fingers exacerbates the pain and is diagnostic of tendon sheath infection. Extensor tendons over the dorsum of the hand are by contrast devoid of sheaths.

Ch 4, p. 77, *Fig 4.47, 4.48, 4.49*

10   A tropical ulcer of the lower limb:

a – true, b – false, c – true, d – true, e – true

A tropical ulcer usually presents with a long history of chronicity and is invariably caused by trivial injury with inoculation of infective organisms. The ulcers are usually punched out with sloping edges which on occasion undermine the surrounding skin (Buruli ulcer). Development of rolled, everted edges in a long-standing ulcer indicates squamous carcinomatous transformation (Marjolin's ulcer). Mycotic ulcers are typically painless and produce pigmented granules.

Ch 4, p. 79, *Fig 4.58*
Ch 6, p. 110–11
Ch 29, p. 393, *Fig 29.25(k), Fig 29.25(m)*

11   Delayed wound healing is associated with:

a – true, b – true, c – true, d – false, e – true

Wound healing is affected by a legion of local and systemic factors. Therefore, there is no 'normal' healing time for a surgical wound. Traumatic wounds are often contaminated and unless wound toilet is meticulous, are susceptible to infection and delayed healing. Poor nutritional status and systemic disease states delay healing.

Ch 4, p. 80–1

12 AIDS defining lesions in patients with seroconversion (AIDS-positive blood test) that are clinically diagnosed are:

a – true, b – false, c – true, d – false, e – false

There are several stages of HIV infection prior to the development of AIDS. Infection with the virus may be asymptomatic or may present with an acute seroconversion illness. AIDS defining illness may be (a) infective: e.g. cerebral toxoplasmosis, pulmonary or oesophageal candidiasis, disseminated mycobacterial and herpes simplex infections and cryptosporidium or cryptococcal related enteritis; or (b) non-infective: e.g. bowel or cerebral lymphoma, Kaposi's sarcoma and multifocal leucoencephalopathy.

Ch 5, p. 86–103, *Fig 5.9, 5.10, 5.17, 5.19, 5.20, 5.21, 5.22, 5.23*

13 Anal warts are:

a – true, b – false, c – true, d – false, e – true

Anal warts are caused by a papilloma virus and usually transmitted during homosexual activity. They are usually multiple and are found in the perianal skin and in the anorectum. They are minimally symptomatic but may cause itching with resultant excoriation of the surrounding skin. They are soft, moist, red, pink or pale exuberant lesions which may grow rapidly and become pedunculated; bleeding is uncommon.

Ch 5, p. 95, *Fig 5.50*
Ch 25, p. 325, *Fig 25.13*

14 Clinical features following ingestion of a corrosive liquid are:

a – false, b – true, c – false, d – true, e – false

Clues to the type of poison ingested are obtained from the history and from objects found in the vicinity of the patient, such as food or liquid remnants, drugs or detergents. Ingestion of corrosive substances produce chemical burns of the mouth, pharynx, oesophagus and/or stomach. The initial burning sensation is caused by the inflammation and ulceration of the lining epithelium. This is followed by a deep-sited dull pain as the visceral wall necroses, with ensuing signs of mediastinal or peritoneal contamination and inflammation.

Ch 7, p. 127–8

15 A sebaceous horn is:

a – false, b – false, c – false, d – false, e – false

Sebaceous cysts are a common clinical finding; occasionally they
may ulcerate, to form a Cock's peculiar tumour, or the contents
of the cyst may gradually escape to build up concretions on the
surface to form a conical sebaceous horn.

Ch 8, p. 139, *Fig 8.34, 8.35, 8.36*

**16 An adult presents with a four-month history of a minimally
symptomatic red, raised, velvety plaque-like lesion involving
the corona and glans of an uncircumcised penis. The lesion is:**

a – false, b – true, c – true, d – true, e – false

Bowen's disease is squamous carcinoma-in-situ which when
involving the penis is referred to as erythroplasia of Queyrat.
It may appear as an encrusted raised red-brown lesion and may
resemble an eczematous plaque. Bowen's disease also occurs in
the vulva where it is frequently multifocal in origin and may
extend into the vagina, the urethra or the anus. It is important to
distinguish this lesion from venereal infections such as granuloma
inguinale, chancroid, lymphogranuloma venereum and syphilis.

Ch 8, p. 140, *Fig 8.38*
Ch 27, p. 354, *Fig 27.26, 27.27*

17 A cutaneous malignant melanoma:

a – false, b – true, c – false, d – false, e – true

Malignant melanomas arise from melanocytes in normal skin and
only a minority develop from pigmented naevi. Malignant change
in a pre-existing naevus is difficult to assess; a change in size,
shape, itchiness or bleeding should arouse suspicion. Satellite
lesions may appear in the surrounding skin or between the
primary lesion and the lymphatic drainage site.

Ch 8, p. 144–5, *Fig 8.51, 8.52, 8.53*

18 A pilonidal sinus:

a – true, b – true, c – true, d – false, e – false

Detached hair, piercing the skin in the web spaces of the hands
(e.g. in hairdressers), in the umbilicus or in the natal cleft
produces a focus of chronic infection that develops into an
abscess and thence into a discharging sinus. Extension is usually
into the surrounding subdermal fat resulting in multiple sinus
formation.

Ch 21, p. 269
Ch 25, p. 326, *Fig 25.14*

19 An umbilical erosion:

a – false, b – false, c – false, d – true, e – false

Umbilical erosions are uncommon and are usually found in the
obese where the umbilicus is 'buried' in the fatty folds of the
abdominal skin. This is conducive to concretions of desquamated
surface epithelium or dirt, or an occasional foreign body
becoming impacted therein, resulting in skin excoriation and
eventual ulceration with a serosanguinous discharge. A pilonidal
sinus of the umbilicus may present similarly with hairs protruding
from the orifice.

Ch 21, p. 269–70

20 Acute appendicitis is:

a – true, b – true, c – false, d – false, e – true

Investigations are rarely required in arriving at a diagnosis of
acute appendicitis. The diagnosis may be difficult in children
and women of child-bearing age due to mesenteric adenitis and
tubo-ovarian lesions respectively producing similar clinical
pictures. Abdominal signs may be obscured by the administration
of narcotic analgesia and repeated clinical examination over the
ensuing hours usually clarifies the diagnosis. In pregnancy, as the
uterus enlarges, the appendix is displaced upwards and may be
situated under the liver near term producing a complex clinical
picture.

Ch 24, p. 304–6

21 A pelvic abscess:

a – false, b – true, c – false, d – true, e – true

A pelvic abscess is the result of an ongoing infective process in the peritoneal cavity. The usual causes are appendicitis, salpingitis and diverticulitis. Fullness or tenderness during rectal or vaginal examination in the presence of a pyrexia and abdominal or bowel symptoms is strongly suggestive of pus in the pelvis. Retro-peritoneal or pre-peritoneal suppuration does not collect in the pelvis but tracks along the fascial planes to points in the flank or groin.

Ch 24, p. 315–17

Section 3

Injuries

1 Diagnostic features of shock in an injured patient include:

a – true, b – false, c – false, d – true, e – true

The clinical diagnosis of shock is based on inadequate organ perfusion and tissue oxygenation, and in identifying the probable cause of shock. Haemorrhage is the most common cause in the injured patient; septicaemia, neurogenic and cardiogenic causes also produce shock; isolated head injuries do not result in shock, whereas, spinal injuries do.

Ch 2, p. 22–3

2 Triage in trauma management is a system for:

a – true, b – false, c – false, d – true, e – false

When receiving and assessing victims of trauma, triage is the sorting of patients based on the severity of their injury and the available resources to provide care. Triage is also performed 'on the field', i.e. at the site of the incident when it is used to allocate patients to appropriate hospitals prior to transportation thereby avoiding inappropriate patient transfers.

Ch 7, p. 115

3 The primary survey of the multiply-injured patient is the:

a – false, b – false, c – false, d – true, e – true

Trauma patients are assessed on the severity of their injuries, the stability of their vital signs and the injury mechanism.
Assessment and management may take place simultaneously and consists of rapid primary evaluation, resuscitation of vital functions followed by a more detailed secondary assessment and the initiation of definitive care. Thus the primary survey identifies the need or otherwise for urgent therapeutic measures.

Ch 7, p. 116

4 The secondary survey of the multiply-injured patient is:

a – true, b – false, c – true, d – false, e – false

The secondary survey of the injured patient does not begin until the primary survey is completed, resuscitation commenced and vital functions reassessed. The secondary survey is a 'head to toe' evaluation of the patient. Each region of the body is examined fully in order to detect any occult injuries or complications of injuries already identified. Thus the potential for missing a significant injury in a multiply injured, unstable, disorientated or unconscious patient is minimized.

Ch 7, p. 119–20

5 A 19-year-old female gymnast fell off the parallel bars and complained of severe neck pain:

a – false, b – false, c – false, d – false, e – true

The patient must be moved strapped to a long spine board with the head and neck immobilized in a collar, head straps and bolsters. Restraints are removed only after exclusion of a spinal injury on adequate plain radiology. Absence of neck muscle spasm or neurological signs of cord injury does not exclude a cervical spinal injury; a minimally displaced vertebral fracture or a dislocation may be unstable requiring only the slightest movement to result in catastrophic cord injury.

Ch 7, p. 116

6 The following clinical findings in a patient suspected of internal injuries calls for urgent resuscitation:

a – true, b – false, c – true, d – true, e – true

Airway obstruction or lung compression are foremost causes of rapid fatality; circulatory failure is second, followed by brain injury. A decreased level of consciousness indicates decreased cerebral oxygenation from respiratory or circulatory compromise, or owing to the direct effect of brain injury. Thus an altered level of consciousness calls for an immediate re-evaluation of the patient's ventilation, perfusion and tissue oxygenation as hypoxaemia compounds a brain injury. Lacerations of the heart or the great vessels in the chest are rapidly fatal but are salvageable if adequate resuscitation permits angiographic evaluation of the injury.

Ch 7, p. 115–21

7 Following a crush injury to the chest:

a – false, b – false, c – true, d – false, e – false

Life-threatening chest injuries identified in the primary survey are: airway obstruction, pneumothorax, flail chest, massive haemothorax and cardiac tamponade. Following immediate management of these conditions the secondary survey attempts to identify the following occult injuries (which are no less life threatening): pulmonary and myocardial contusions, tracheobronchial and aortic disruptions, and oesophageal and diaphragmatic injuries. These injuries may not be immediately recognizable and a high index of clinical suspicion is required to confirm the diagnosis, with appropriate imaging studies.

Ch 7, p. 116–17
Ch 19, p. 249, *Fig 19.23, 19.24*

8 In a six-year-old child sustaining hot water scalds to the chest and abdomen, the:

a – true, b – true, c – true, d – true, e – false

A child with such an injury is invariably distressed as are his or her carers. Emotional and physical support is best provided in hospital. It is inadvisable to discharge a child with a greater than 10% superficial or partial thickness burn, due to the increased risk of infection, and the need for fluid replacement and prophylactic antibiotic therapy. Paralytic ileus may also develop curtailing immediate oral feeding.

Ch 7, p. 122–4, *Fig 7.2, 7.4*

9 In a patient with a penetrating chest wound and cardiac tamponade there is:

a – true, b – false, c – true, d – false, e – true

Cardiac tamponade is commoner in penetrating than in blunt chest injuries. As the pericardial sac fills with blood the classic Beck's triad (venous pressure elevation, arterial pressure drop and muffled heart sounds) is diagnostic. Pulsus paradoxus (a decrease in systolic arterial pressure during inspiration in excess of 10 mmHg) and Kussmaul's sign (a rise in venous pressure with inspiration when breathing spontaneously) are also characteristic of tamponade. The diagnosis is confirmed by pericardiocentesis.

Ch 7, p. 120

10 A 50% body surface burn in a conscious and orientated 70-year-old patient requires:

a – true, b – false, c – false, d – true, e – true

Extensive surface burns and increasing age are poor prognostic indicators of survival. This patient appears to have sustained a non-survivable burn injury and may have only a few hours to live. Extensive resuscitation or specific treatment measures may only be instituted at the request of the patient or relative following counselling. Adequate analgesia and privacy with loved ones and/or a priest should take priority.

Ch 7, p. 123, *Fig 7.3*

11 A burn injury to an extremity:

a – true, b – false, c – true, d – false, e – true

A partial thickness surface burn is exquisitely tender and moist with blebs unlike deep burns which are relatively dry and insensitive. Rapid assessment of the extent of a burn injury is required to commence analgesic, fluid and antibiotic therapies. Once an inhalation injury is excluded, the burn areas are mapped out, indicating whether full or partial thickness, and the percentage of the surface involved calculated.

Ch 7, p. 122–5, *Fig 7.6*

12 In a young adult with suspected smoke-inhalation injury:

a – false, b – false, c – true, d – true, e – false

In a patient with a burn injury to the face the possibility of airway injury is present. Although the larynx protects the trachea and bronchi from direct heat and smoke, they are extremely susceptible to obstruction from inflammatory oedema and mucus plugs produced by the injury. There are few immediate signs of impending respiratory failure following smoke inhalation. It is therefore imperative to identify early signs of respiratory distress such as throat irritation, coughing and breathlessness. Arterial blood gas measurement reflects the state of gaseous exchange at the alveolar level.

Ch 7, p. 123

13 In a machine operator who sustained high tension electrical burns to his hand and buttock:

a – false, b – true, c – true, d – true, e – true

High tension electrical injury may precipitate ventricular arrhythmias requiring immediate cardio-pulmonary resuscitation. Tissue damage along the passage of the electric charge in the body may occur leading to muscle necrosis and myoglobinuria. The resulting oedema may compromise adjacent structures and a compartment syndrome may develop and must be recognized early.

Ch 7, p. 125

14 In a cutaneous burn injury:

a – true, b – false, c – false, d – false, e – false

First degree burns result from over-exposure to the sun or momentary contact with a hot surface and are characterized by erythema, pain and the absence of skin blebs. Second degree burns involve the epidermis and superficial layers of the dermis; they are caused by severe sunburn, hot liquids and flash burns. In third degree burns both the epidermis and the dermis are destroyed, and a variable amount of underlying tissue. Second and third degree burns may result in considerable tissue swelling and intra-vascular fluid loss.

Ch 7, p. 122–4, *Fig 7.4*

15 Frost bite of an extremity may be diagnosed by:

a – false, b – true, c – true, d – false, e – true

Frost bite is due to freezing of tissue with intracellular ice crystal formation and microvascular stasis leading to cell death. Cold injuries in temperatures above freezing may lead to 'trench foot' or 'immersion foot' where there is a history of cold and dampness leading to skin maceration and superficial necrosis.

Ch 7, p. 126, *Fig 7.7*

16 A pensioner was rescued from an unheated dwelling suffering from severe hypothermia and frostbite to both feet:

a – true, b – false, c – false, d – true, e – false

Cardiac arrhythmias occur at core temperatures below 32°C and asystole may supervene below 28°C; rewarming of the patient may reactivate the heart. It is therefore essential to rewarm the patient before confirming cardiac arrest. Hypothermia is associated with pulmonary hypertension and left heart failure and may produce electro-mechanical dissociation with absent pulses. The line of demarcation between viable and non-viable tissue usually regresses following rewarming.

Ch 7, p. 126, *Fig 7.7, 7.8*

17 In a 'blow-out' fracture of the orbit:

a – false, b – false, c – false, d – true, e – true

Despite the presence of periorbital haematoma and swelling with conjunctival ecchymosis and chemosis, orbital injuries rarely cause ocular damage. Enophthalmos and diplopia are found when there is a significant displacement of the eye into the orbital floor fracture; entrapment of an extra-ocular muscle in the fracture may also produce double vision. Supra- or infra-orbital nerve injury may result in paraesthesia of the forehead or cheek.

Ch 12, p. 182

18 A cervical spine injury:

a – true, b – false, c – true, d – false, e – true

A patient with an injury above the clavicle or a head injury resulting in loss of consciousness should be suspected of an associated cervical spinal injury. Therefore injudicious neck movements during examination may exacerbate an occult vertebral injury. Unstable vertebral injuries when present may be detected in the immobilized patient, by plain radiology that delineates the cervical spine from the atlanto-occipital joint to the upper surface of the 1st thoracic vertebra.

Ch 30, p. 407–8, *Fig 30.23*

19 A 50-year-old lumberjack severed the sciatic nerve in the buttock in an accident involving a chain-saw; the clinical presentation is:

a – true, b – false, c – true, d – true, e – false

Sciatic nerve injuries are uncommon but may occur during posterior dislocation of the hip and hip replacement surgery. Sciatic nerve root compression is a complication of lumbar disc prolapse or degeneration; paralysis of the flexors and extensors of the foot results in an equinus deformity with patchy cutaneous anaesthesia.

Ch 31, p. 416–17

20 In a tibial fracture:

a – true, b – false, c – false, d – false, e – false

Limb fractures are often missed in the multiply injured patient. Long bone fractures when occurring alone are usually obvious from the symptoms and local signs. In a compound fracture there is communication of the fracture haematoma with the exterior. The presence of arterial pulses distal to the fracture with normal sensation does not exclude a developing compartment syndrome. An associated neurovascular injury is excluded by normal limb sensation and palpable pedal pulses. Plain radiography of the injured limb must be obtained in two planes and should include the joints above and below the fracture as an associated injury to an adjacent joint is occasionally present.

Ch 32, p. 419–20, *Fig 32.2*

21 In a closed fracture of a long bone:

a – false, b – false, c – true, d – false, e – false

Fractures of the humerus and femur usually produce deformity, swelling, crepitus and abnormal movement. In the forearm and leg, where the two long bones are bound by interosseous ligaments, fracture of one bone may not exhibit many of the above signs as it is splinted by its companion. Neurovascular injury may occur either from direct injury or from compression in unyielding fascial compartments. A compartment syndrome manifests as pain greater than expected, exacerbated by stretching the muscles; absence of a distal pulse is a late sign as capillary flow to the affected muscles is compromised long before arterial flow is affected.

Ch 32, p. 419–20

22 There is swelling, pain and bruising of the arm and elbow in an eight-year-old boy following a fall on his outstretched hand:

a – true, b – true, c – false, d – false, e – true

A supracondylar fracture of the arm in a child may be associated with injury to the neurovascular bundle due to the forward displacement of the humeral shaft, compromising limb viability. Radial pulse, hand sensation and finger movements must be monitored during the examination. Plain radiology with lateral views identifies the injury and avoids unnecessary manipulation.

Ch 35, p. 449, *Fig 35.6, 35.7*

23 A 19-year-old man self-inflicted a laceration to his left wrist with division of the median nerve; the presentation is:

a – false, b – true, c – false, d – false, e – false

The ulnar and median nerves supply all intrinsic muscles of the hand and are liable to injury in slashing wounds to the wrist. The long flexor tendons, and the radial artery and vein may also be injured. The clinical picture is likely to be complex and the integrity of the structures in the carpal tunnel may require assessment under anaesthesia. The radial nerve becomes a purely cutaneous nerve to the dorsum of the hand. The ulnar nerve supplies the muscles of the hypothenar eminence and the finger abductors and adductors. The median nerve supplies the muscles of the thenar eminence. Paralysis of all small muscles produces a claw hand (*main-en-griffe*).

Ch 35, p. 451–2

24 In a man with a pelvic ring disruption injury sustained in a road traffic accident there was blood staining at the urethral meatus. The following are required to evaluate his injury:

a – false, b – false, c – false, d – true, e – true

Disruption of the pelvic ring is a sequela to a crush injury to the pelvis. It results in internal bleeding from retro-peritoneal and/or pelvic visceral lacerations leading to hypovolaemic shock. Severe pain with skin bruising around the pelvis and signs of peritoneal irritation are a good indicator of visceral injury. Resuscitatory measures should commence before haemodynamic changes become manifest. The urethra and the urinary bladder, particularly if the latter was full, are the most susceptible to injury and imaging studies are required for confirmation when the patient is haemodynamically stable.

Ch 37, p. 461–3, *Fig 37.1, 37.3*

25 **Following the resolution of pain and swelling of an injured knee, a football player found the knee 'gave way' when weight bearing; the probable diagnosis is a:**

a – false, b – false, c – true, d – false, e – false

The cruciate ligaments provide antero-posterior stability of the knee joint. Following a rupture of a cruciate ligament, the stability in one of these directions is lost and has to be compensated for by quadriceps or gastrocnemii muscle action in steadying the joint. This is adequate for most sedentary activities.

Ch 38, p. 478–9, *Fig 38.16*

26 **A cricketer complains that his left knee suddenly locked whilst playing; he would:**

a – true, b – true, c – false, d – true, e – false

Acute knee injuries are caused by linear or rotational forces being imparted on a limb that is firmly implanted on the ground. True locking of the knee is the inability to fully extend the joint which may then 'unlock' either spontaneously or following manipulation. Meniscal and anterior cruciate tears produced by injury or degenerative changes, and loose bodies which are fragments from articular cartilage or menisci as a result of attritional damage, all produce locking. Arthroscopic inspection is required to identify the cause.

Ch 38, p. 478–9

27 **A rugby player suffered severe pain and swelling over the anterior aspect of the knee on kicking a ball; he may present with the following:**

a – true, b – true, c – true, d – false, e – true

Collateral or cruciate ligaments are torn in sporting activities resulting in tenderness over the damaged ligament and an acute effusion or bleeding into the joint. Avulsion of the tibial tuberosity is seen in adolescents whilst a 'distraction' fracture of the patella during sudden forceful extension is unusual. Medial ligamentous or meniscal injuries are frequently associated with a torn anterior cruciate ligament. Ligamentous injuries of the knee are difficult to diagnose and an examination under anaesthesia is required to determine the extent of joint instability.

Ch 38, p. 478–80, *Fig 38.16, 38.18*

28 The radiological findings that are suggestive of child abuse are:

a – false, b – false, c – true, d – true, e – false

There is a disturbing increase in the prevalence of child abuse in contemporary society. Increasing family pressures brought about by social, economic and cultural changes of modern-day life are contributory. Repeated attendances to the accident and emergency departments of one or more hospitals with injuries or non-specific ill-health, or departing before being seen, should alert the clinician to the possibility of deliberate harm to the child. Social services have clear guidelines for investigating and protecting the child.

29 The signs of physical abuse in the elderly are:

a – false, b – false, c – false, d – true, e – false

When there is increasing difficulty in obtaining suitable residential care for the elderly, more and more old people are compelled to live with unsuitable 'carers' lacking in awareness of, and a commitment to, their needs. Ill-treatment is usually concealed by the sufferers due to their emotional and/or economic dependence on their carers. Physical evidence must be looked for when there is a history of repeated injuries or accidents at home.

Head, face and neck

1 Oral candidiasis was found in a 79-year-old woman admitted with an unrelated systemic illness; the diagnosis is suggested by the following:

a – false, b – false, c – false, d – false, e – false

Oral candidiasis appears as a sticky white membrane over the tongue or buccal mucosa and the scrapings when examined microscopically suspended in normal saline show the fungal filamentous structure. Leukoplakia is a white lesion on the surface of the mucous membrane as is erythroplasia (red, raised mucosal lesions) both of which have a predilection to malignancy.

Ch 1, p. 12, *Fig 1.42*
Ch 13, p. 192–3, 197, *Fig 13.25, 13.38*

2 A 59-year-old woman presents with an asymptomatic swelling in the right supra-clavicular fossa; the possible diagnoses are:

a – true, b – true, c – true, d – false, e – true

Supraclavicular lymph nodes act as the watershed to lymphatics draining the neck, chest wall and breast, and communicate with the axillary, mediastinal and coeliac lymph nodes. Thus occult cancers arising in these regions may present as palpable deposits in the root of the neck.

Ch 3, p. 52, *Fig 3.14*
Ch16, p. 215–8, *Fig 16.2, 16.5*

3 A pulsatile lump on the side of the neck in a 83-year-old man would suggest the following:

a – true, b – true, c – false, d – false, e – false

Carotid artery aneurysms are usually due to arteriosclerotic disease, resulting in the loss of the elastic lamina. Carotid body tumours are closely applied to the carotid bifurcation and may give rise to a pulsatile lesion. Rarely a false aneurysm may develop following arterial puncture; this is caused by bleeding into the perivascular space producing a pulsatile haematoma. Mycotic and syphilitic aneurysms are rare in the neck.

Ch 3, p. 52, *Fig 3.16*

4 Acute raised intracranial pressure:

a – true, b – true, c – false, d – true, e – true

Any expanding intracranial lesion produces a raised intracranial pressure. Tumours produce a very gradual increase in pressure in contrast to intracranial haemorrhage. Mass lesions stretch the oculomotor nerve producing pupillary changes on that side. Later, herniation of the brain through the tentorium cerebelli or the foramen magnum leads to rapid loss of brain stem activity.

Ch 9, p. 156

5 An epidural haemorrhage is distinguished from a subdural haemorrhage by a:

a – true, b – true, c – false, d – false, e – true

The characteristic findings in an extradural haematoma are loss of consciousness followed by a period of lucidity and a further relapse into unconsciousness, with the development of a hemiparesis and a dilated fixed pupil as late signs. During the lucid interval the patient usually has a severe localized headache and may feel drowsy. Subdural haematoma is associated with tearing of dural veins and/or cortical arteries with an underlying cerebral contusion or laceration. The patient remains unconscious and a decrease of two or more GCS points during the period of assessment indicates rapid deterioration of cerebral function requiring immediate remedial measures.

Ch 9, p. 157–8

6 An adult is admitted semi-conscious making incomprehensible noises and localizes painful stimuli; he is, however, unable to respond to verbal commands. He has a GCS score of:

a – false, b – false, c – true, d – false, e – false

The Glasgow Coma Scale measures spontaneous eye, verbal and motor responses, and those following verbal and painful stimuli. The score reflects cortical activity and scores of 8 or less signify severe deficit. Cerebral function may deteriorate rapidly after the initial trauma due to progressive compression or a fall in oxygenation; a GCS 'flow chart' enables early identification of such deterioration.

Ch 9, p. 157–8

7 A young woman admitted as an emergency with a diagnosis of a subarachnoid haemorrhage would manifest the following:

a – true, b – true, c – false, d – true, e – false

Primary or spontaneous subarachnoid haemorrhage is most often due to a ruptured Berry aneurysm of the circle of Willis; less commonly arteriovenous malformations or blunt head trauma are causative factors. Occasionally Berry aneurysms prior to rupture give rise to pressure symptoms on the III, IV, V and VI cranial nerves producing a squint, double vision or facial pain. Meningeal irritation follows rupture, producing severe occipital headache, vomiting, dizziness, convulsions and/or coma. Neck stiffness develops after a few hours with positive Kernig and Babinski responses. Hemiplegia may develop if the bleeding is sufficient to produce a space occupying lesion. The important differential diagnosis is bacterial meningitis.

Ch 9, p. 159

8 A 56-year-old man developed a right-sided third cranial nerve palsy as a result of a Berry aneurysm of the right posterior communicating artery; he may present with:

a – true, b – true, c – false, d – true, e – false

Features of a complete oculomotor nerve palsy are ptosis, with the eye turned outwards and downwards, and pupillary dilatation and loss of accommodation, due to loss of the parasympathetic mediated pupillary reflex, resulting in blurring of vision on the same side.

Ch 9, p. 160, *Fig 9.23*

9 Brain death in a comatose patient may be diagnosed:

a – false, b – false, c – true, d – true, e – true

Tests for brain stem death are: – pupils fixed and dilated; – no corneal reflex; – no gag reflex; – no vestibulo-ocular reflexes; – no motor response to pain stimuli within the cranial nerve distribution; – no respiratory movements on stimulating the respiratory centre (apnoea testing). Severe hypothermia produces cardiorespiratory arrest which may be reversed on rewarming. Drug intoxication also produces cardiorespiratory arrest which may be reversed by resuscitation and organ support with detoxification. Decerebrate and decorticate rigidity signify brain stem lesions that are irreversible.

Ch 9, p. 159

10 In unilateral facial nerve injury there is:

a – false, b – true, c – true, d – true, e – false

Complete transection of the facial nerve as it emerges from the stylomastoid foramen results in flaccid paralysis of all muscles of facial expression on that side. When the injury is to one or more branches, e.g. during parotid surgery, the palsy is limited to the distribution of those affected branches. Paralysis of the eyelids produces conjuctival irritation, and that of the buccinator and orbicularis oris cause difficulty with eating.

Ch 9, p. 161, *Fig 9.26, 9.27, 9.28*

11 Carcinoma of the maxillary antrum in a 46-year-old wood worker typically presents with:

a – true, b – true, c – true, d – true, e – true

These tumours are uncommon and are squamous cell carcinomas. Patients may present with a persistent nasal discharge, a blocked nasal passage or an enlarged neck node. Antroscopy and mucosal biopsy are required for confirmation. Carcinoma of the hard palate and sarcoma of the upper jaw present similarly.

Ch 10, p. 164–5
Ch 12, p. 180, *Fig 12.33*
Ch 13, p. 196, *Fig 13.30*

12 A patient with Bell's palsy has paralysis of the:

a – false, b – true, c – false, d – false, e – true

This is an idiopathic lower motor neurone lesion of the facial nerve. Other causes of facial nerve paralysis include cerebello-pontine angle tumours, Ramsay Hunt syndrome, basal skull fracture, parotid gland infiltration (sarcoid, lymphoma, amyloid), mononeuritis multiplex (diabetes mellitus, systemic vasculitides) and iatrogenic injury.

Ch 10, p. 168

13 A four-year-old girl was found to have a hearing loss in one ear six months after an acute ear infection. A diagnosis of 'glue ear' was made and the clinical findings were:

a – false, b – false, c – true, d – true, e – true

Conductive deafness in a child is usually due to chronic otitis media (glue ear) resulting from an unresolved middle ear infection. Chronic suppurative otitis media presents with hearing loss, an intermittent or persisting discharge and may be associated with developmental or behavioural problems. It is characteristically painless and predisposing conditions include adenoidal inflammation, cleft palate and barotrauma.

Ch 11, p. 172–3, *Fig 11.16*

14   A patient with hearing loss:

a – true, b – true, c – true, d – false, e – false

The degree of hearing disability is dependent on the extent of the deafness and whether only one ear is affected. A history of noise exposure is found with some occupations. A genetic predisposition to deafness may be present. Middle ear infection is a common cause of conductive deafness and a discharge or inflammation of the ear-drum must be visualized. Drugs such as gentamicin, propranolol, frusemide, aspirin, quinine and cisplatin are ototoxic.

Ch 11, p. 172–3

15   A patient suffering from vertigo:

a – true, b – false, c – true, d- true, e – false

A patient with vertigo has a sensation of movement of self with respect to the surroundings or vice versa. Vertigo may be labyrinthine or central nervous in origin. It is important to ascertain the severity and length of each episode and its frequency. Paroxysmal positional vertigo is triggered by head movements and is of abrupt onset and transient. Recurrence of vertiginous attacks, fluctuating hearing loss and tinitus are features of Ménière's syndrome. Benign paroxysmal positional vertigo is of abrupt onset but transient and is triggered by head movements.

Ch 11, p. 173

16   A painful red eye is characteristic of:

a – true, b – false, c – true, d – true, e – true

Pain, redness, photophobia and watering are found in keratitis, anterior uveitis/iritis, scleritis and episcleritis. In bacterial conjunctivitis the eye is red, itchy and sticky. Acute glaucoma also causes a painful red eye which feels hard and an early diagnosis is essential to preserve sight.

Ch 12, p. 177–80, *Fig 12.17, 12.23, 12.25, 12.26*

17   A stone in the submandibular salivary gland duct presents with:

a – true, b – true, c – true, d – false, e – false

Calculus obstruction of a salivary duct may lead to glandular infection from stasis. Tumours of the submandibular salivary gland are rare and present as swellings and include epidermoid carcinoma, leukaemias and melanoma. Exfoliative cytology is helpful in screening and a trans-oral biopsy is essential for establishing a diagnosis.

Ch 15, p. 213–14, *Fig 15.9, 15.10, 15.13, 15.14*

18   An 18-year-old man presents with an asymptomatic midline swelling in the front of his neck; the possible lesions are:

a – true, b – true, c – false, d – false, e – false

Thyroid swellings are midline structures unless there is asymmetric enlargement of one lobe. Dermoid cysts are superficial midline lesions usually found in the lower half of the neck. Lymph nodes, branchial cysts and cystic hygromas are laterally placed and are situated below the ear, the last being present at birth.

Ch 16, p. 217–21, *Fig 16.6, 16.18*

19   A thyroglossal cyst:

a – false, b – true, c – false, d – true, e – false

A thyroglossal cyst is a remnant of the thyroglossal duct; it is a midline structure in the front of the neck and is distinguished from a solitary nodule arising from the isthmus of the thyroid by its movement upward on protrusion of the tongue. It is susceptible to infection and may present as an abscess over the thyroid cartilage; discharge on to the surface results in a non-healing sinus.

Ch 17, p. 225–6, *Fig 17.7, 17.8, 17.9*

20 A meningo-myelocoele in a neonate may present as:

a – false, b – true, c – true, d – true, e – true

Defective closure of the vertebral column (spina bifida et occulta) is one of the most severe neural defects compatible with prolonged life. The clinical presentation varies from the occult type with few clinical signs, to a completely open spine. In spina bifida cystica, the protruding sac over the back may contain meninges (meningocoele), spinal cord (myelocoele) or both (meningomyelocoele). Spina bifida is commonly sited in the lower thoracic, lumbar and sacral regions. When the spinal cord or nerve roots are involved there is a varying degree of paralysis below the involved level. Since the paralysis is present during fetal development, skeletal development may be affected with coexisting disorders, such as kyphosis, arthrogryphosis, dislocated hips and club foot. The paralysis may also involve the bladder and anal sphincters.

Ch 30, p. 402–3, *Fig 30.15, 30.16*

Endocrine and breast

1 In a patient presenting with Graves' disease the following serum parameters would be raised:

a – true, b – false, c – false, d – true, e – true

Primary thyrotoxicosis involving the entire functioning thyroid gland (Graves' disease) is caused by abnormal thyroid stimulating antibodies; thus TSH secretion is suppressed by the high levels of circulating thyroid hormones. The goitre is vascular and a bruit may be auscultated over the upper poles.

Ch 2, p. 36–7, *Fig 2.23, 2.24, 2.25, 2.26*

2 Thyrotoxicosis is characterized by:

a – true, b – true, c – false, d – true, e – false

The patient is usually a young female and the condition may be familial. The thyroid is usually moderately and diffusely enlarged and soft, and a bruit may be heard. The patient feels hot and the skin is warm and moist due to peripheral vasodilatation. Weight loss may be a feature despite increased food intake. Sleep tachycardia is present and palpitations may be troublesome. Fine hand tremor with general hyperkinesia and increased bowel motility may be present. Eye signs are usual. Anxiety is common and psychiatric disturbance rare. Menstrual irregularity and infertility may occur.

Ch 2, p. 36–7, *Fig 2.25, 2.26*
Ch 17, p. 223

Answers and comments

3 Myxoedema is characterized by:

a – true, b – false, c – false, d – false, e – true

There is a gradual change in personality coupled with physical characteristics of facial puffiness, coarse skin, a large tongue and a gruff voice. There is hair loss, constipation and menorrhagia. Mental apathy, drowsiness and, rarely, depressive illness and dementia may be simulated. Cardiac enlargement and abnormal heart sounds suggest pericardial myxoedema. Deep tendon reflexes may show a slow recovery phase – a useful diagnostic sign.

Ch 2, p. 38, *Fig 2.27, 2.28*
Ch 17, p. 225

4 Characteristic dermatological features of Cushing's syndrome include:

a – false, b – true, c – true, d – false, e – true

There is truncal obesity with 'moon facies' and prominent supraclavicular and dorsal cervical fat pads. The skin is thin and atrophic with purple striae due to stretching and exposure of dermal capillaries. The skin, therefore, bruises easily and heals poorly. The extremities are thin due to muscle wasting. Oligomenorrhoea, osteoporosis, glucose intolerance and psychological disturbances are common.

Ch 2, p. 39, *Fig 2.31, 2.32*

5 A 29-year-old woman with biochemical evidence of anterior pituitary gland overactivity would present with:

a – false, b – true, c – true, d – false, e – true

The adult features of pituitary-dependent Cushing's syndrome due to increased production of glucocorticoids is characteristic. Young adult females are predominantly affected. The secretory tests used to confirm the diagnosis are:

– plasma cortisol levels and diurnal variation;
– 24-hour urinary free cortisol excretion;
– overnight low-dose dexamethasone suppression test.

These assist in distinguishing Cushing's syndrome from adrenal cortical hyperfunctioning tumours and ectopic ACTH-secreting tumours.

Ch 2, p. 39, *Fig 2.31, 2.32, 2.33*

6 In Addison's disease:

a – true, b – true, c – false, d – false, e – true

Features of Addison's disease are fever, vitiligo, nausea, anorexia, vomiting and abdominal pain, with diarrhoea or constipation. Joint and back pain and myalgia may be present, along with impotence and amenorrhoea. Trauma or infection may precipitate an adrenal crisis and the patient may go into shock. Patients are therefore encouraged to wear a bracelet identifying the disease, the current medication and advice on therapy if taken ill.

Ch 2, p. 40, *Fig 2.36, 2.37, 2.38*

7 A goitre:

a – false, b – true, c – false, d – true, e – false

A goitre is any swelling of the thyroid gland and lies within the investing layer of the deep cervical fascia. Enlargement of the thyroid gland bears no relationship to its functional status. Clinical assessment of a goitre is rarely adequate as its functional state must be assessed biochemically and by isotope uptake. Fine needle aspiration cytology is useful in evaluating functionally inactive areas of the gland which may be cystic or neoplastic; haemorrhage into a cyst or a tumour undergoing central necrosis may produce pain.

Ch 17, p. 223, *Fig 17.1, 17.2*

8 Papillary carcinoma of the thyroid:

a – false, b – true, c – true, d – false, e – false

Papillary carcinoma accounts for 60% of all thyroid malignancies and is prognostically the most favourable of the thyroid cancers. It metastasizes late to cervical lymph nodes but has a good prognosis despite nodal spread. The diagnosis is confirmed by fine needle aspiration cytology or exploratory surgery and frozen section histology. Occasionally the primary in the thyroid gland is impalpable with a solitary deposit in an enlarged lymph node, the so-called 'lateral aberrant thyroid'.

Ch 17, p. 224

9 A 41-year-old woman with a medullary carcinoma of the thyroid gland may present with:

a – false, b – true, c – true, d – true, e – true

Medullary (C-cell) carcinoma presents as a firm to hard swelling of one or both thyroid lobes. Spread to cervical lymph nodes as well as blood-borne spread may occur and the likely sites for distant metastases must be examined. Serum calcitonin levels are raised in medullary carcinoma, with normal serum calcium levels.

Ch 17, p. 224–5, *Fig 17.3*

10 A solitary nodule of the thyroid gland in a 32-year-old woman:

a – false, b – false, c – true, d – false, e – false

The solitary thyroid nodule is a common presentation of thyroid pathology. The majority are cysts readily confirmed on ultrasound scanning; they are usually asymptomatic unless haemorrhage produces pain due to rapid expansion. In the solid nodule malignancy must be excluded. Selenium-methionine radio-isotope scan or fine needle aspiration cytology may aid in the diagnosis.

Ch 17, p. 225, *Fig 17.4, 17.5*

11 A 49-year-old man was diagnosed to have parathyroid overactivity; he would exhibit the following:

a – true, b – false, c – false, d – false, e – true

Increased production of parathyroid hormone is due to parathyroid hyperplasia and adenoma leading to increased serum calcium and alkaline phosphatase levels from bone resorption and excretion of phosphate in the urine. Patients may present with loin pain due to calcium stone formation in the kidneys.

Ch 17, p. 226

12 Parathyroid gland(s):

a – false, b – true, c – false, d – false, e – true

Tetany in hypoparathyroidism is due to increased neuromuscular excitability. Latent tetany may be demonstrated by Chvostek's or Trousseau's sign. The severity of the tetany is generally related to the degree of hypocalcaemia. Mild hypercalcaemia is usually asymptomatic and is an incidental finding on routine screening. Circumoral paraesthesia may be the first symptom. Anorexia, nausea, weakness and abdominal pain along with thirst and polyuria follow. Tonic contractions are present in severe hypocalcaemia and may become generalized. Long-term complications are urolithiasis and nephrocalcinosis, with radiological features of bone disease.

Ch 17, p. 226–7, *Fig 17.10, 17.11*

13 Advanced breast cancer may present with:

a – true, b – false, c – true, d – true, e – true

A breast tumour exceeding four centimetres in size is locally advanced. There is an increased likelihood of spread to regional lymph nodes and distant metastases. Tethering of the tumour to overlying skin heralds eventual ulceration, and fixity to the pectoral fascia indicates chest wall involvement. Inflammatory carcinoma is rare and may present with erythema and induration without a palpable lump.

Ch 18, p. 230–4, *Fig 18.6, 18.7, 18.8, 18.11*

14 A carcinoma of the breast in a 61-year-old woman is clinically staged as $T_2 N_2 M_1$; this implies:

a – false, b – false, c – false, d – false, e – true

A malignant clinical diagnosis requires staging to document the extent of the disease. Breast imaging with fine needle aspiration cytology may be required to confirm the diagnosis of the primary lesion. Fine or core needle biopsy of palpable axillary nodes is required to confirm axillary spread. Distant spread may be assessed by liver and bone scans.

Ch 18, p. 231–4, *Fig 18.6, 18.7, 18.8, 18.13*

15 An ulcerating lesion over a previously healthy mastectomy scar in a 63-year-old woman suggests:

a – false, b – false, c – true, d – false, e – false

Local recurrence of breast cancer following ablative surgery has an incidence of 5% over 10 years. Modern adjuvant chemo- and radiotherapy following surgery have low complication rates and skin breakdown is a rarity. Local recurrence following adequate treatment, though distressing does not adversely influence survival. A second primary (metachronous tumour) arising following breast-conserving surgery for cancer is usually found away from the previous scar. They are more often detected by the patient and brought to the attention of the clinician.

Ch 18, p. 233–4, *Fig 18.14*

16 Nipple discharge:

a – false, b – true, c – true, d – false, e – true

Nipple discharge may be associated with a palpable lump in the nipple–areolar complex. Manually expressing the secretion may identify the number of ducts involved. Mammography and ultrasonography may not detect a small intraduct papilloma or a carcinoma. Cytology should therefore be obtained on a blood-stained discharge.

Ch 18, p. 234–5, *Fig 18.17*

17 The following types of nipple discharge in a 35-year-old woman are associated with:

a – false, b – true, c – false, d – false, e – false

Nipple discharge is a common presenting symptom of breast disease and the clinical association of a discharge with an underlying pathology assists in arriving at a diagnosis. Duct papillomas and carcinomas are the only lesions that produce a blood-stained discharge and alert the clinician to the underlying cause, even in the absence of a palpable lesion. Serous or greenish discharge is associated with duct ectasia and a purulent discharge occurs when a retro-areolar abscess discharges through the nipple.

Ch 18, p. 234, *Fig 18.12, 18.16, 18.17*

18 In a lactating 34-year-old woman presenting with pain, swelling and reddening of the right breast:

a – true, b – true, c – true, d – true, e – true

An inflammatory swelling of the breast in a woman of child-bearing age does not exclude an inflammatory carcinoma, even during lactation. However, an inflammatory swelling in a peri- or post-menopausal woman must be regarded with a high index of clinical suspicion. Breast imaging may not be helpful in the absence of a mass. Aspiration needle cytology or core biopsy is required to confirm the diagnosis.

Ch 18, p. 236–7, *Fig 18.19, 18.21*

19 A secretory focus that is situated away from the nipple–areolar complex of a lactating breast suggests:

a – true, b – false, c – true, d – false, e – false

Accessory breasts and nipples are anatomic aberrations situated along the milk line that extends from the axilla across the chest to the pubis. A mammary fistula is the result of an abscess involving a lactiferous duct discharging on to the surface and the tract being maintained by duct secretion.

Ch 18, p. 236–7, *Fig 18.20*

20 A 30-year-old woman complaining of back pain, tiredness and paroxysmal headaches was found on isotope scanning to have a phaeochromocytoma. The clinical presentation includes:

a – false, b – true, c – true, d – false, e – false

Adrenal tumours are diagnosed on imaging and biochemical parameters. The clinical manifestations are those of overproduction of catecholamines from the adrenal cortex.

Ch 23, p. 289, *Fig 23.24*

Chest and spine

1 A psoas abscess:

a – true, b – true, c – false, d – true, e – false

Tuberculosis is the usual cause of a 'cold' abscess at the groin. Tuberculosis of the dorsal spine produces destruction of adjacent vertebral bodies by caseation leading to collapse and spinal angulation. The paravertebral abscess tracks down deep to the psoas fascia and points in the groin. There is usually a long history of poor health and backache. Compression of the nerve roots may produce paraesthesia and weakness of the legs and compression of the cord results in paraplegia.

Ch 4, p. 65, *Fig 4.6*
Ch 30, p. 406, 30.21

2 Clinical indications of an inhalation injury are:

a – true, b – false, c – true, d – true, e – true

Airway compromise due to smoke inhalation in a patient extracted from a fire must be looked for, as the supraglottic airway is relatively unprotected and is very susceptible to inflammatory oedema from exposure to heat or fumes. Dyspnoea and central cyanosis are late signs of respiratory injury requiring urgent ventilatory support.

Ch 7, p. 124

3 Carbon monoxide poisoning in a patient rescued from a fire is suggested by:

a – true, b – true, c – true, d – false, e – false

Carbon monoxide poisoning must be presumed in victims of fires or gas leaks in enclosed spaces. The characteristic cherry-red skin coloration is rare and arterial pO_2 measurements do not reliably predict the extent of carbon monoxide poisoning. Mental disturbance or alterations in consciousness occur from hypoxia when there are significant carbon monoxide levels in the blood.

Ch 7, p. 124

4 A pneumothorax in a 36-year-old woman is:

a – false, b – true, c – false, d – false, e – true

Symptoms from a spontaneous pneumothorax depend on its size and the extent of any underlying lung disease. With a small collection of air physical signs may be absent but as the former increases auscultatory findings become manifest. Mediastinal shift becomes evident in a large or a tension pneumothorax but hypoxaemia may be absent and signs of respiratory distress a late manifestation in a previously healthy young adult.

Ch 19, p. 241-2, *Fig 19.3*

5 Empyema of the pleural cavity:

a – false, b – true, c – false, d – false, e – true

Empyema thoracis is a complication of progressive lung suppuration. Percussion is dull with reduced vocal fremitus and vocal resonance over the collection in the pleural cavity; pus may be loculated giving rise to characteristic radiological features. As the collection expands mediastinal shift becomes clinically obvious with progressive reduction in functional lung volume.

Ch 19, p. 242–4, *Fig 19.9*

Answers and comments

6 Progressive respiratory failure is characterized by:

a – false, b – true, c – true, d – true, e – false

The need to use the accessory muscles of respiration for normal breathing is characteristic of chronic obstructive airway disease which is an irreversible generalized airway obstruction associated with chronic bronchitis and/or emphysema. The disease may begin early in life in smokers though significant symptoms and disability do not manifest until late adult life. Mild ventilatory abnormalities may be present long before the onset of clinical symptoms. The presenting symptom is exertional dyspnoea that is gradually progressive or precipitated by an acute respiratory infection. A consistent physical finding is slowing of forced expiration; auscultatory findings are, however, inconsistent and variable.

Ch 19, p. 242–4, *Fig 19.10*

7 Cough, haemoptysis and weight loss over a five-month period in a 65-year-old man suggest:

a – false, b – true, c – true, d – false, e – false

The potentially serious significance of blood in the sputum is generally known in societies where lung cancer is the leading cause of cancer deaths in adults. Patients may not volunteer this information out of anxiety or fear and must be specifically asked. When purulent sputum is mixed with blood pulmonary suppuration is the presumed diagnosis; this may be primary as in bronchiectasis or empyema thoracis, or secondary as with an inhaled foreign body or an obstructing bronchial tumour. Smoking habits should also be enquired into as cigarette smoking is the single most important risk factor in chronic lung disease and lung cancer.

Ch 19, p. 242–6, *Fig 19.12*

8 **A 48-year-old cigarette smoker with a history of recurrent chest infections presented with a chronic cough and breathlessness. Bronchial carcinoma may be excluded if:**

a – false, b – false, c – false, d – false, e – false

Most primary lung cancers are endobronchial and a persistant cough is invariable. The sputum from an ulcerated bronchial tumour is usually not excessive but contains inflammatory exudate and may be blood-streaked; significant bleeding due to vascular tumour erosion is rare. Bronchial narrowing by the tumour leads to adventitious breath sounds and eventually to segmental collapse; infection in that segment may present with malaise, fever, chest pain and loss of weight.

Ch 19, p. 245–7, *Fig 19.12, 19.17*

9 **A patient with an acute episode of angina pectoris exhibits:**

a – false, b – false, c – true, d – false, e – false

The diagnosis of coronary artery disease is dependent on an accurate history. The chest pain of angina is characteristically provoked by exertion, cold weather or occasionally by emotional stress. It occurs during rather than after exercise. The pain of myocardial infarction is more severe and is accompanied by nausea, vomiting and profuse sweating; it is unrelieved by nitroglycerine. The pain of aortic dissection is similar and radiates through the chest to the back with circulatory collapse.

Ch 20, p. 255–6, *Fig 20.1*

10 **A 37-year-old woman with a diagnosis of aortic stenosis presents with:**

a – true, b – false, c – false, d – true, e – false

Heart murmurs are caused by abnormal blood flow patterns associated with valvular defects or anaemia. The character of a murmur is an unreliable guide to its origin. However, loud, coarse murmurs are associated with valvular narrowing and soft, blowing murmurs with valvular incompetence. The position over the chest where the murmur is loudest and the direction of its radiation enables the identification of the valvular lesion. Haemodynamic murmurs are soft, are present in both systole and diastole and do not radiate.

Ch 20, p. 261–4, *Fig 20.7*

Answers and comments

11 A 61-year-old man with stenosis of the mitral valve may present with:

a – true, b – false, c – true, d – true, e – false

The patient may give a history of rheumatic fever and present with constricting chest pain and breathlessness. There is a low rumbling diastolic murmur with signs of pulmonary oedema; right ventricular failure may be a consequence of pulmonary hypertension with dependent oedema.

Ch 20, p. 261–4, *Fig 20.7*

12 A neonate was found to cough and choke on feeds; chest auscultation revealed bilateral adventitious sounds. He may have:

a – true, b – true, c – true, d – false, e – true

It is advised that the first feed of a newborn should be water and not milk to test the swallowing reflex and the integrity of the upper GI tract. Choking at birth should warn of a possible developmental anomaly and be investigated by the passage of a paediatric feeding tube with aspiration of gastric contents. Failure of gastric intubation should lead to oesophageal imaging with a water-soluble contrast medium.

Ch 26, p. 332–3, *Fig 26.5, 26.6*

13 Scoliosis of the spine is diagnosed by:

a – false, b – true, c – false, d – true, e – true

Scoliosis is commonest in adolescence where it is idiopathic and usually unnoticed if < 20° (Cobb's angle). Progressive angulation occurs in curves of > 30° which are conspicuous and associated with backache or respiratory symptoms when there is angulation of the rib cage. Emotional overlays to symptoms may occasionally be encountered in adolescents.

Ch 30, p. 398–9, *Fig 30.4, 30.6*

14 A 49-year-old man complains of chronic low backache that is progressive and exacerbated by physical activity. He may be suffering from:

a – true, b – true, c – true, d – true, e – true

Chronic low back pain over the age of 40 is a common complaint that usually originates from (a) degenerative disease of the spine, e.g. bony ankylosis, arthritis or stenosis of the spinal canal, (b) defects in the articular facets, e.g. spondylosis and spondylolysthesis or (c) intervertebral disc degeneration. The straight leg raising test distinguishes nerve root pain from mechanical back pain; plain spinal radiology assists in the diagnosis.

Ch 30, p. 399, *Fig 30.5*
Ch 30, p. 404–5, *Fig 30.17, 30.18, 30.19*

15 In cervical spondylosis:

a – true, b – false, c – true, d – true, e – false

Cervical spondylosis is part of a spectrum of acute and chronic neuromuscular disorders affecting the neck muscles and/or the nerve roots. Symptoms range from neck stiffness to painful muscle spasms of the posterior neck and occiput, to acute root pain with sensorimotor defects in the distribution of C6, C7 and C8 nerve roots. Pain is the most frequent symptom and radiates from the back of the neck or base of the skull to the shoulder or scapula, with occasional radiation down the arm. Deep tenderness and muscle spasm may be elicited over the cervical spinous processes. There may be evidence of muscle wasting and diminished reflexes along the nerve root involved.

Ch 30, p. 404–5

16 A 17-year-old boy presents with a 10-week history of back pain. Examination revealed a dorsal spinal deformity and associated muscle spasm:

a – true, b – true, c – true, d – false, e – true

Tuberculous spondylitis (Pott's disease of the spine) is seen mainly in children with variable presenting symptoms. Nagging back pain is present and may radiate to the abdomen. A prominent and tender spinal process may be palpable due to anterior wedging of adjacent vertebral bodies. A paraspinal abscess may track up or down to present in the supraclavicular fossa or the groin. Cord compression by an abscess in the dorsal spine produces symptoms varying from minor loss of bladder and/or bowel control to sudden and irreversible paraplegia. Plain radiology reveals anterior destruction of vertebral bodies and the intervening discs, with wedging and a space occupying surrounding abscess.

Ch 30, p. 406, *Fig 30.21*

17 A 32-year-old woman with lateral prolapse of the C8–T1 intervertebral disc presents with:

a – false, b – false, c – false, d – true, e – true

The disc prolapse is usually precipitated by a sudden twisting movement of the neck resulting in severe pain and muscle spasm. The pain may radiate over the shoulder and down the upper arm. There may be paraesthesia and weakness in the upper limb down to the fingers.

Ch 30, p. 404–5

18   A 36-year-old man with suspected spinal cord compression requires the following procedures for diagnostic confirmation:

a – true, b – false, c – true, d – true, e – false

Spinal cord or root compression is caused by osteoarthritic or degenerative changes of the spine or by spinal tumours. Nerve root pain may be uni- or bilateral with limb paraesthesia, weakness or spasticity. The Brown–Sequard syndrome is found in hemi-cord dysfunction caused by extradural tumours; there is ipsilateral tactile and contralateral pain and temperature sensory loss below the level of the lesion. Complete cord paralysis occurs with untreated spinal tumours with cessation of all sensory and motor function distally.

Ch 30, p. 404–5, *Fig 30.18, 30.20*

19   A 65-year-old long-term male cigarette smoker presents with mild facial oedema, hoarseness, moderately distended neck veins, left-sided Horner's syndrome and pain radiating down his left arm. These suggest:

a – true, b – true, c – true, d – true, e – false

Late symptoms of bronchial carcinoma include hoarseness, weakness, localized chest pain and weight loss. Peripherally situated tumours may invade the pleura with serosanguinous pleural effusions. Horner's syndrome results from invasion of the cervical sympathetic chain; infiltration of the chest wall and the brachial plexus may occur with apically situated tumours (Pancoast syndrome). Superior vena caval obstruction and recurrent laryngeal nerve palsy are produced by extension of the tumour from mediastinal lymph nodes. Intrapulmonary spread of cancer may result in lymphangitic carcinomatosis with cor pulmonale. Paraneoplastic (extra-pulmonary) manifestations may produce neurological, endocrine, haematological and musculo-skeletal lesions.

Ch 31, p. 412–13, *Fig 31.2*

20   Injury to the long thoracic nerve of Bell presents as:

a – false, b – false, c – true, d – false, e – true

The long thoracic nerve of Bell is a motor nerve supplying the serratus anterior muscle which stabilizes the shoulder girdle during flexion and forward movement of the arm. Damage to the nerve may occur during axillary lymph node dissection and results in an unsightly deformity of the back during pushing. Scapular winging is also found in paralysis of the trapezius muscle.

Ch 31, p. 412–14, *Fig 31.1*

Section 7

Abdomen

1 A tender upper abdominal swelling in a 56-year-old woman with normal vital signs and a serum amylase of 900 IU suggests:

a – true, b – false, c – true, d – true, e – false

In acute pancreatitis severe abdominal pain and tenderness restrict clinical assessment of the abdomen, though guarding and rigidity may not be present except when the disease is fulminating or haemorrhagic. Skin ecchymoses may be present in the flank and/or the umbilicus one or two days following the onset. Bowel sounds are scanty or absent and abdominal distension occasional. The presence of a palpable abdominal mass reflects extensive inflammation or the onset of complications such as abscess or pseudocyst formation.

Ch 2, p. 40, *Fig 2.35*
Ch 21, p. 267–8, *Fig 21.3, 21.4*

2 In an eight-year-old Asian child with massive hepatosplenomegaly the causative disease states are:

a – true, b – true, c – false, d – false, e – true

Progressive enlargement of the liver and spleen is found in veno-occlusive disease, portal hypertension, childhood leukaemias and tropical parasitic infections. Acute infections produce a tender liver or spleen due to the rapid inflammatory stretching of the capsule. Infarction of splenic tissue occurs in marked splenomegaly producing pain and occasionally an audible bruit. A purpuric rash and mucosal bleeding suggests hypersplenism.

Ch 6, p. 109, *Fig 6.5*

3 In acute necrotizing pancreatitis:

a – false, b – true, c – true, d – true, e – false

Acute necrotizing pancreatitis presents with severe upper abdominal pain radiating to the flanks and the back, with anorexia, nausea, vomiting and prostration. There is tenderness and guarding with reduced or absent bowel sounds. Signs of pancreatic haemorrhage may manifest as bruising in the umbilicus (Cullen's sign) or the flanks (Grey Turner's sign). Hypovolaemic shock may occur due to fluid loss into the 'third space' or haemorrhage into the gland. Endotoxic shock is a late manifestation of pancreatic necrosis and secondary infection.

Ch 21, p. 267–8, *Fig 21.3, 21.4*
Ch 24, p. 303

4 Abdominal aortic aneurysms:

a – false, b – true, c – true, d – false, e – true

The presence of an expansile, pulsatile abdominal mass is diagnostic of an aortic aneurysm. Pain on presentation or tenderness on palpation are ominous signs suggesting a recent increase in size. An ultrasound scan measures the transverse diameter and an aneurysm exceeding six centimetres is associated with a significant incidence of leakage and rupture.

Ch 21, p. 268, *Fig 21.5*
Ch 24, p. 313, *Fig 24.12*
Ch 28, p. 376, *Fig 28.34*

5 The physical findings that assist in the diagnosis of inguinal herniae are:

a – true, b – false, c – false, d – false, e – false

Examining a groin hernia with a view to making a diagnosis is regarded as an essential skill. The positions of the internal and external inguinal rings in relation to the two bony landmarks – the pubic tubercle and the anterior superior iliac spine – assist in the identification of the defect in the inguinal canal.

Ch 22, p. 271–4, *Fig 22.1, 22.2, 22.3*

Abdomen

6 An umbilical hernia is:

a – true, b – false, c – false, d – false, e – true

Umbilical hernia is common in the neonate and gradually retracts into the abdominal wall as the child matures. It is usually asymptomatic and strangulation is rare. It is more prevalent in African children.

Ch 22, p. 275, *Fig 22.8*

7 Hepatomegaly is:

a – true, b – false, c – false, d – true, e – false

Liver enlargement is a clinical finding when the liver edge descends below the costal margin. The commonest causes are fatty infiltration, venous congestion and viral hepatitis. In early cirrhosis the liver enlarges due to an inflammatory reaction before shrinking as fibrosis replaces the liver parenchyma. Neoplastic change in the cirrhotic liver may progress to an enlarged and palpable liver. Jaundice implies a defect in bilirubin metabolism or secretion, and liver enlargement without jaundice may not reflect functional impairment.

Ch 23, p. 284, *Fig 23.17*

8 A 73-year-old woman with a pancreatic cancer may present with:

a – true, b – true, c – true, d – true, e – true

Symptoms of pancreatic cancer are non-specific; jaundice may be present when the tumour involves the pancreatic head; the tumour is usually impalpable but in obstructive jaundice the liver is enlarged and a distended gall bladder may be palpable (Courvoisier's law). Splenic venous thrombosis leading to splenomegaly is unusual. A high index of clinical suspicion is needed to diagnose pancreatic cancer at an early stage with appropriate imaging studies.

Ch 23, p. 288

9 A patient with Peutz–Jeghers syndrome may:

a – false, b – true, c – true, d – true, e – true

This is a familial hamartomatous polyposis affecting the small bowel and occasionally extending to the large bowel. It is usually diagnosed early in life by the tell-tale pigmentation of the lips and oral mucosa. Patients are generally asymptomatic though bowel obstruction progressing to an intussusception may be caused by a large polyp. Neoplastic change is known to occur when hamartomatous polyps are present in the colon.

Ch 23, p. 290, *Fig 23.25*

10 Common presentations of Crohn's disease include:

a – false, b – true, c – false, d – true, e – true

Due to similarities of presentation of inflammatory bowel disease, malabsorption syndromes and chronic infective diarrhoeas reliance is placed on the history in arriving at a clinical diagnosis. In inflammatory bowel disease the acute presentation is with fever, malaise, mucoid and/or bloody diarrhoea, abdominal pain and tenderness; recurrent and subacute episodes may be associated with bowel obstruction, abscess or fistula formation and nutritional debility. Transmural bowel inflammation causes adhesions, fissuring and ulceration which may progress to fistulation into an adherent viscus or onto the abdominal or perianal skin.

Ch 23, p. 290, *Fig 23.26, 23.27*

11 Causes of severe rectal bleeding are:

a – true, b – true, c – false, d – false, e – false

Bright red blood per rectum suggests a bleeding source not far removed from the anus and is usually confined to the rectum and sigmoid colon. Profuse bleeding from the more proximal colon can also present similarly. Bowel cancers do not bleed profusely and tumours of the proximal colon usually present with melaena. The most frequent cause of severe bleeding is diverticular disease. All patients with rectal bleeding require proctoscopy, sigmoidoscopy, colonoscopy and/or a barium enema examination, to rule out an occult neoplasm.

Ch 23, p. 292–3, *Fig 23.30, 23.32*

12 A 33-year-old stock-market trader complains of severe upper abdominal pain relieved by eating with a marked periodicity over a nine-month period; other probable symptoms are:

a – true, b – false, c – false, d – false, e – true

Dyspeptic symptoms with their characteristic periodicity and relief from alkali ingestion are characteristic of peptic ulcer disease. Pain and vomiting in a chronic gastric ulcer may be food-induced. The finding of haematemesis and/or melaena is diagnostic and an endoscopy or barium studies is required for confirmation.

Ch 24, p. 300, *Fig 24.1*

13 A 34-year-old doctor returning from working in a refugee camp in Eastern Europe develops features suggestive of an acute liver abscess; these are:

a – true, b – false, c – true, d – true, e – true

Pyogenic liver abscess usually presents with fever, loss of appetite, weakness and upper abdominal discomfort. The liver may not be palpable, jaundice is unusual and leukocytosis may be absent; there is shortness of breath from a pleural effusion. Amoebic liver abscess usually follows an episode of amoebic dysentery when the patient was resident in an endemic area. Liver imaging determines the presence, the location and the number of abscesses.

Ch 24, p. 303–4

14 A 26-year-old woman was referred with a suspected diagnosis of acute appendicitis; the positive findings are:

a – true, b – false, c – true, d – false, e – true

The diagnosis of acute appendicitis in women of child-bearing age is difficult, due to acute gynaecological lesions that may present similarly. Anorexia and nausea, with foul breath and a furred tongue, are expected findings; abdominal pain that shifts after a few hours from being central or generalized to the vicinity of the inflamed appendix is characteristic. Pelvic lesions that may mimic acute appendicitis are acute salpingitis, ruptured ectopic pregnancy and a twisted or ruptured ovarian follicle.

Ch 24, p. 304–6, *Fig 24.5*

15 Small bowel obstruction:

a – true, b – false, c – true, d – true, e – true

Mechanical bowel obstruction is due to intraluminal, transluminal or extraluminal organic lesions. Prolonged obstruction eventually leads to paralytic ileus from peristaltic efforts to overcome the blockage. Ileus may also be due to enteric or systemic toxins. Unrelieved bowel obstruction may lead to bowel ischaemia due to the intraluminal pressure exceeding the perfusion pressure; this predisposes to the transudation of bowel pathogens into the peritoneal cavity and eventual perforation.

Ch 24, p. 307–8, *Fig 24.7*

16 A 28-year-old male AIDS sufferer presents with non-specific abdominal symptoms and is found to have a colonic intussusception on CT scanning; the clinical findings are:

a – true, b – true, c – true, d – true, e – true

Symptoms of colonic obstruction are insidious in onset and there may be spurious diarrhoea in incomplete obstruction. The commonest causes in the adult are faecal impaction, diverticular disease and colonic carcinoma. In AIDS with gastrointestinal manifestations, intussusception may be caused by hyperplasia of bowel lymphatic tissue, bowel lymphoma or Kaposi's sarcoma. A contrast-enhanced abdominal CT scan assists in establishing an early diagnosis.

Ch 24, p. 309–10, *Fig 24.9*

17 A neonate presents with projectile vomiting following feeds and his mother noticed a transient firm lump in his abdomen soon after. The probable diagnoses are:

a – false, b – false, c – false, d – true, e – false

Projectile vomiting is a characteristic symptom of pyloric stenosis and rarely of duodenal atresia or an annular pancreas. Vomiting must be distinguished from regurgitation of feeds due to oesophageal anomalies or a poorly developed swallowing reflex.

Ch 26, p. 333–4

18   An infant with congenital megacolon presents with:

a – true, b – true, c – true, d – false, e – false

The functional obstruction of Hirschsprung's disease may cause enterocolitis secondary to bacterial overgrowth. This may result in a fulminant diarrhoea with rapid loss of fluid and electrolytes which, in toxic megacolon, may be rapidly fatal. Early clinical diagnosis of megacolon in a child is based on a history of chronic constipation, abdominal distension and failure to thrive; confirmation is by mucosal biopsy.

Ch 26, p. 335–6, *Fig 26.7, 26.8*

19   A 79-year-old man with an adenocarcinoma (hypernephroma) of the kidney may present with:

a – true, b – true, c – true, d – true, e – true

Haematuria is the usual presenting symptom, occasionally with clot colic. There may be loin discomfort or pain and the patient may have noticed a loin swelling. A rapidly developing varicocoele (usually on the left) is a striking but a rare finding due to the tumour obstructing the testicular vein on that side. Atypical presentation may result from neoplastic deposits in bone or lung. There may be pyrexia, anaemia or rarely a polycythaemia, the last due to the production of erythropoietin by the tumour. Diagnostic confirmation is by renal imaging.

Ch 27, p. 342, *Fig 27.7, 27.8*

20   Renal colic is:

a – true, b – false, c – true, d – true, e – false

Renal calculus disease presents as renal colic, and defects in calcium, purine or cysteine metabolism are common underlying causes. Calculi in the ureter produce colic which may be referred to the groin; they usually pass spontaneously but occasionally require endoscopic extraction. Calculi retained in the pelvicalyceal system may enlarge causing renal damage (stag-horn calculus).

Ch 27, p. 343–4, *Fig 27.9, 27.12*

Section 8

Pelvis

1 Transillumination is positive in the following scrotal lesions:

a – true, b – false, c – true, d – false, e – true

Transillumination determines the lucency of a fluid collection or a soft tissue swelling in the scrotum. Testicular or epididymal pathology may not be readily palpable in a fluid-filled scrotum while ultrasound scanning is usually diagnostic of these lesions. However, the diagnosis of testicular torsion and orchitis must be made clinically, in view of the urgency of treatment for the former.

Ch 3, p. 53, *Fig 3.17*
Ch 27, p. 359–62, *Fig 27.42, 27.44, 27.46*

2 An indirect inguinal hernia:

a – true, b – true, c – false, d – true, e – false

Inguinal hernias are common; the symptoms may be diverse but the diagnosis should be straightforward provided the basic steps of examination are followed. Small impalpable hernias are, however, difficult to confirm and greater reliance is placed on the history. Defects lateral to the internal ring are uncommon, they include interstitial and Spigelian hernias.

Ch 22, p. 271–3, *Fig 22.2, 22.4*

3 A femoral hernia:

a – true, b – true, c – true, d – false, e – false

Femoral hernias are notoriously difficult to diagnose as they are frequently impalpable and a cough impulse is absent. The incidence of strangulation is significantly higher than in inguinal hernias and a Richter-type hernia is not unusual. Tenderness with a history of a transient swelling and/or pain in the area of the femoral triangle is usually sufficient indication for surgical exploration.

Ch 22, p. 274–5, *Fig 22.5, 22.6*

4 A patient with early carcinoma of the rectum may present with:

a – true, b – true, c – false, d – false, e – false

Carcinoma of the rectum, unlike more proximal colonic cancers, usually presents early due to the resulting anorectal discomfort or pain and the associated tenesmus, mucoid or bloody discharge or loss of continence. Digital rectal examination detects virtually all anal and rectal cancers and the diagnosis is confirmed by proctoscopy and biopsy.

Ch 23, p. 292, *Fig 23.30*

5 Haemorrhoids:

a – true, b – false, c – false, d – true, e – true

External haemorrhoids are observed on perianal inspection whilst internal haemorrhoids require proctoscopic visualization. Fresh rectal bleeding must not be attributed to haemorrhoids without investigating the colon for other causes, namely, colorectal cancer. Diverticular disease frequently coexists with haemorrhoids in the older age group and may account for the bleeding. Anal pain is caused by a thrombosed pile and presents as a tender firm lump at the anal verge.

Ch 25, p. 321, *Fig 25.2, 25.3, 25.4*

6 Rectal prolapse:

a – true, b – true, c – true, d – false, e – true

Rectal prolapse may be mucosal (partial) or involve the entire rectal wall (complete). Mucosal prolapse is common in children and is self-limiting; in adults it is usually associated with third degree haemorrhoids or a lax anal sphincter. Complete prolapse is due to pelvic floor laxity from child birth, pelvic surgery or ageing; it may also be associated with utero-vaginal prolapse.

Ch 25, p. 325, *Fig 25.11*

7 A 59-year-old man with prostatic symptoms is diagnosed on digital rectal examination to have a prostatic cancer; the positive findings include a:

a – false, b – true, c – true, d – false, e – true

Prostatic cancer may only be diagnosed clinically when it is locally advanced and has breached the capsule (TNM stage T3 or T4) or from clinically obvious metastatic deposits. Prostatic symptoms are investigated by urinary flow studies and prostate specific antigen (PSA) titres. Significantly raised levels require transrectal ultrasonography which detects and stages the disease. A transrectal core biopsy or a transurethral prostatectomy provides material for histological grading.

Ch 27, p. 345–6, *Fig 27.14*

8 Chronic urinary retention is:

a – false, b – false, c – false, d – true, e – true

Bladder outflow obstruction in infancy and childhood is due to bladder neck hypertrophy (Marion's disease) or posterior urethral valves; in the young adult the usual cause is inflammatory urethral stricture; later in life prostatic hyperplasia and neurogenic bladder are the leading causes.

Ch 27, p. 345–6, *Fig 27.14*

9 The urinary bladder is:

a – false, b – false, c – false, d – false, e – false

Chronic urinary obstruction is usually due to prostatic hyperplasia or urethral stricture in the adult and bladder neck hypertrophy and posterior urethral valves in the infant. It is usually painless and progressive bladder distension with increasing volumes of residual urine leads to recurrent urinary infection and diverticula formation. Acute retention is extremely painful and is usually due to prostatic obstruction or 'clot colic' with the patient presenting as an emergency.

Ch 27, p. 345–6, *Fig 27.14, 27.15, 27.16*

10 A 62-year-old woman under surveillance for transitional cell carcinoma of the bladder, treated by cystoscopic resection, develops symptoms suggestive of a recurrence; they include:

a – false, b – true, c – false, d – false, e – false

In a patient previously treated for a bladder neoplasia, painless haematuria should be regarded as indicating a recurrence of the lesion; bleeding, however, is rarely profuse. Bladder tumours may also present with recurrent urinary tract infections. Pelvic or perineal pain is a late symptom and suggests tumour extension to the pelvis.

Ch 27, p. 346, *Fig 27.15*

11 A nine-year-old Asian boy was found to have a vesical stone on plain abdominal radiology. His clinical presentation would include:

a – true, b – true, c – true, d – true, e – true

Primary bladder stones usually originate in the kidney and on reaching the bladder grow in size. Secondary stones are formed in the presence of urinary stasis, infection or foreign bodies. Frequency is the earliest symptom; pain occurs at the end of micturition and may be referred to the tip of the penis or vulva; the passage of a few drops of blood at the end of micturition is also characteristic and both these symptoms are caused by the stone abrading the vascular trigone.

Ch 27, p. 346, *Fig 27.16*

12   A 37-year-old woman with a clinical diagnosis of chronic pyelonephritis is likely to present with:

a – true, b – true, c – true, d – false, e – true

Chronic pyelonephritis is also referred to as reflux nephropathy due to its association with vesico-ureteric reflux and women under the age of 40 years form the majority of sufferers. Systemic symptoms are non-specific, and include lassitude, malaise, anorexia and nausea. Dull loin or low back pain may also be present but occasionally they may be overlooked until renal function is significantly compromised. Hypertension is present in 40% of cases and develops slowly and is associated with long-standing disease. Clinical findings are a low grade fever and a normochromic anaemia; pus cells in the urine are indicative of a bacterial infection which suggests the diagnosis.

Ch 27, p. 347

13   A 27-year-old man is diagnosed to have chronic prostatitis; the clinical presentation is:

a – true, b – true, c – true, d – true, e – true

Intermittent fever, body-ache and malaise are common constitutional symptoms of prostatitis. A urethral discharge following prostatic massage may provide the causative organism. Prostatic abscess is a rare complication of acute prostatitis and a rectal examination reveals an enlarged, very tender, hot and perhaps a fluctuant prostate.

Ch 27, p. 351

14   An inflammatory urethral stricture in a 29-year-old man presents with:

a – true, b – true, c – true, d – true, e – true

The early symptoms are difficulty in voiding with poor urinary stream, dribbling and frequency. The youthfulness of most sufferers distinguishes urethral stricture from prostatic enlargement. In an established stricture the surrounding fibrous scarring may be palpable. Diagnosis is confirmed on urethroscopy or by urethrogram.

Ch 27, p. 354, *Fig 27.25*

15 A painful chronic genital ulcer is:

a – true, b – false, c – false, d – true, e – true

A history of sexual exposure is of importance in the evolution of a genital ulcer. Genital herpes may start with local irritation, erythema and papule formation, leading to blistering and ulceration. Later, a crust forms as the ulcer heals. A syphilitic ulcer also heals when the disease progresses to the secondary stage. Genital warts are characteristic in appearance and rarely ulcerate.

Ch 27, p. 355–6, *Fig 27.29, 27.30, 27.31, 27.32*

16 A 21-year-old man presented with a six-month history of testicular symptoms; a clinical diagnosis of a testicular tumour was made on the following:

a – true, b – true, c – true, d – false, e – false

Testicular swelling, heaviness and less frequently pain are the presenting symptoms of testicular cancer. There may be a history of maldescent. There is loss of testicular sensation and the testis is enlarged and may feel irregular and heavy; a secondary hydrocoele may be present. Occasionally the presentation is due to metastatic disease with abdominal or lumbar pain, an abdominal mass or rarely a supraclavicular mass. A plain chest radiograph may reveal pulmonary metastases in testicular teratomas.

Ch 27, p. 357, *Fig 27.37, 27.38*

17 A vaginal hydrocoele is:

a – true, b – true, c – true, d – false, e – false

A hydrocoele is invariably painless and, except in the rare complete hydrocoele in infancy, is confined by the testicular tunics to the scrotum. Ultrasonography may be required to delineate the testis from a surrounding hydrocoele, particularly in a young man, to exclude an associated testicular neoplasm.

Ch 27, p. 358, *Fig 27.39*
Ch 27, p. 360, *Fig 27.42, 27.43*

18 Testicular torsion in a 15-year-old boy:

a – false, b – false, c – true, d – true, e – false

Twisting of the testis on its cord spontaneously or following strenuous activity may result from incomplete attachment of the epididymis to the testis or to the mesorchium. Immediate symptoms of torsion are severe localized pain, nausea and vomiting, followed by scrotal swelling and fever. Torsion must be distinguished from inflammatory conditions within the scrotum, testicular trauma and tumour. Immediate surgical relief is essential to prevent testicular atrophy.

Ch 27, p. 358–9, *Fig 27.40*

19 Iliac vein thrombosis in a previously healthy 36-year-old-woman:

a – false, b – false, c – true, d – true, e – false

The usual presentation is a low grade pyrexia and variable swelling of the lower limb(s). Clinical signs, like symptoms, may be minimal, necessitating careful examination for traces of peripheral oedema and tenderness in the calf or medial aspect of the thigh. The diagnosis is confirmed by ultrasonic imaging or venography. A rise in the D-dimer titre in the peripheral blood is suggestive of deep venous thrombosis. Venous occlusion is produced by progression of the thrombosis, and leads to a painful, swollen and deeply dusky limb (phlegmasia cerulea dolens); venous stasis eventually leads to gangrene.

Ch 29, p. 384–6, *Fig 29.3, 29.4, 29.5, 29.6*

20 In a male neonate with complete ectopia vesicae, the clinical features are:

a – true, b – true, c – true, d – true, e – true

This congenital defect is produced by the incomplete development of the infra-umbilical part of the anterior abdominal wall and that of the anterior bladder wall. Thus the mucosa of the posterior bladder wall and part of the trigone protrudes through the defect. Efflux of urine from the exposed ureteric orifices may be observed. The pubic bones are poorly developed and do not meet in the midline. The umbilicus is usually absent and there may be associated paraumbilical and groin hernias.

Section 9

Limbs

1 An inability to extend the fingers is caused by:

a – false, b – true, c – true, d – false, e – true

A flexion deformity of the hand may be caused by contractures from ischaemic or traumatic injury to the forearm, wrist or hand or arthritic damage to the joints. Upper motor neurone lesions also produce flexion contracture of the hand as the flexors are stronger than the extensors.

Ch 1, p. 10, *Fig 1.30*
Ch 36, p. 457, *Fig 36.9*

2 A seven-year-old girl with stunted growth and bowing of the legs:

a – false, b – true, c – true, d – false, e – true

The earliest physical sign in childhood rickets is craniotabes (reduced mineralization of the skull) followed by enlargement of the epiphyseal plates of the long bones, noticeable at the costochondral junctions at the wrists and ankles. Weight bearing bends the long bones causing the rare partial fracture. Pigeon chest deformity is an occasional finding and Harrison's sulcus is formed by the diaphragmatic pull on the soft rib cage.

Ch 2, p. 43, *Fig 2.44*
Ch 32, p. 425, *Fig 32.15, 32.16*

Answers and comments

3 Diabetic ulcers of the foot:

a – true, b – true, c – false, d – true, e – false

Atherosclerotic occlusive disease has a high incidence in diabetes and affects distal limb arteries. A diabetic foot ulcer is the result of critical ischaemia, diabetic neuropathy and infection introduced by minor trauma; it may progress to cellulitis, abscess formation, osteomyelitis or gangrene. Neuropathic and arteriopathic features are present in diabetic ulcers which are found on pressure points of the heel, metatarsal heads and toes and are characteristically painless. Marked skin atrophy in diabetes may predispose to ulceration over the shin with reddish-brown plaques with central ulceration (necrobiosis lipoidica diabeticorum).

Ch 3, p. 56–8, *Fig 3.23, 3.24, 3.25, 3.27, 3.28, 3.29*
Ch 28, p. 372, *Fig 28.23, 28.24, 28.25, 28.26, 28.27*
Ch 29, p. 393, *Fig 29.25*

4 The clinical findings in a patient presenting with an ingrowing toe-nail are:

a – false, b – false, c – true, d – true, e – false

The symptoms from an ingrowing toe-nail vary from minor discomfort to suppuration of the entire nail bed with the nail virtually lifting off the bed. Wearing of shoes with narrowed fronts and raised heels is the commonest cause.

Ch 4, p. 79–80, *Fig 4.59*

5 Dry gangrene of an extremity is characterized by:

a – false, b – true, c – false, d – false, e – false

Gangrene in a limb may present as either 'dry' or 'wet'. The latter is caused by venous or lymphatic occlusion during the period of vascular compromise. Waterlogged dead tissue progresses rapidly to putrefaction with lethal septic complications. In dry gangrene arterial occlusion is present in the absence of outflow compromise; venous and lymphatic channels remain collapsed and there is little retained tissue fluid; sepsis is therefore minimal.

Ch 28, p. 367–71, *Fig 28.9, 28.10*

6 Intermittent claudication:

a – false, b – false, c – true, d – true, e – true

Claudication is due to peripheral vascular disease and its severity is indicated by the distance walked before limb muscle pain halts further progress. Symptoms are more severe when walking uphill but the patient is usually able to continue walking after intermittent rests. Exercise improves the claudication distance by opening up collateral vessels and improving the circulation to the foot. Following exercise on the treadmill, foot pulses that were palpable at rest may disappear. Approximately 1 in 10 claudicants progress to severe limb ischaemia, when postural changes and venous guttering appear.

Ch 28, p. 369, *Fig 28.14, 28.15*

7 Ischaemic foot ulceration:

a – true, b – false, c – false, d – true, e – true

Rest pain is the dominant symptom of ischaemic ulceration which is the result of critical ischaemia in peripheral vascular disease. Initially there is inflammation and reddening of the skin with surrounding trophic skin changes. Ulceration with loss of skin and subcutaneous tissue exposes underlying tendons, joints and bone. In diabetes, an associated peripheral neuropathy leads to painless ulceration.

Ch 28; p. 370–2, *Fig 28.16, 28.17, 28.18, 28.19, 28.20, 28.21, 28.22*

8 Raynaud's phenomenon of the hands is:

a – true, b – true, c – false, d – true, e – true

Raynaud's phenomenon is characterized by intermittent attacks of blanching or cyanosis accompanied by numbness and tingling followed by a burning sensation and pain in the digits; it is usually precipitated by exposure to cold or emotional stress. The condition may be a primary vasospastic disorder (Raynaud's disease) or secondary to associated conditions such as atherosclerosis or scleroderma.

Ch 28, p. 376–7, *Fig 28.35*

9 Varicose veins of the lower limb:

a – true, b – true, c – false, d – true, e – true

Lower limb varices are dilated and tortuous superficial veins due to incompetent valves linking them to the deep venous system. The cause may be familial or secondary to deep vein thrombosis. There is segmental venous hypertension with extravasation of tissue fluid leading to trophic skin changes, with ulceration and bleeding.

Ch 29, p. 387–9, *Fig 29.10, 29.11, 29.12, 29.13, 29.15, 29.16*

10 Lymphoedema of the lower limb:

a – false, b – false, c – false, d – true, e – false

Primary lymphoedema may be congenital or may occur during puberty or later. It is usually found in women with an asymptomatic swelling of the foot, leg or the entire limb. It is worse in warm weather or after prolonged dependency. The oedema is diffuse producing a typical mound of swelling on the dorsum of the foot (or hand) and is usually only partially pitting; this becomes less obvious with the passage of time, due to subcutaneous fibrosis and skin changes. Secondary lymphoedema is commonly caused by infection entering through the foot. The onset is sudden with fever, rigors and a red, hot swollen leg. There is lymphangitis and groin lymphadenitis. The latter distinguishes it from acute thrombophlebitis. Secondary lymphoedema also arises from surgical ablation of regional lymph nodes or from neoplastic infiltration.

Ch 29, p. 394–6, *Fig 29.26, 29.27, 29.28*

11 A 36-year-old woman complains of progressive pain and stiffness in her lower back, with pain radiating down the right buttock and thigh over a four-month period; more recently she experienced pins and needles sensation in the calf and foot. These symptoms are characteristic of:

a – true, b – false, c – true, d – true, e – true

Back pain with signs of nerve root compression generally suggests intervertebral disc degeneration or prolapse. Osteophyte formation with nipping of the nerve roots or nerve root injury from fractures of the lumbar vertebral body may produce a similar picture. Space occupying spinal lesions (cauda equina syndrome) may affect bladder and bowel control as well.

Ch 30, p. 397–402, *Fig 30.2, 30.3, 30.4, 30.5, 30.6*

12 A febrile nine-year-old boy gives a two-week history of pain and swelling in the region of his left knee:

a – true, b – true, c – true, d – false, e – false

Osteomyelitis is a clinical diagnosis and treatment should follow immediately to forestall extension of the disease with bone destruction. Radiological signs of metaphyseal mottling or periosteal new bone formation are usually delayed for two weeks or more. Early signs of localized erythema, induration and tenderness over the bony shaft suggest periostitis which precedes suppuration; malnutrition and anaemia frequently coexist.
In pyomyositis, there is inflammation followed by suppuration of skeletal muscle and may present similarly. Childhood bone tumours are rare but may also have similar presentations.

Ch 32, p. 423–4, *Fig 32.11, 32.12, 32.13*

13 In Paget's disease of the tibia:

a – false, b – true, c – true, d – true, e – false

Paget's disease of the bone is generally asymptomatic and is usually an incidental finding. The warmth, hyperaemia, thickening and bowing of the bone are characteristic of advanced disease in the older age group where this disease is usually found. Due to increased bone vascularity and shunting a high output cardiac failure may also be present. Pathological fracture may occur due to loss of structural stability despite the sclerosis and thickening. Osteogenic sarcoma is a rare complication.

Ch 32, p. 424, *Fig 32.14*

14 A patient with a primary tumour of the femur may present with:

a – true, b – true, c – true, d – true, e – false

Most primary bone tumours are firm or hard swellings. Localized pain is suggestive of rapid growth and the swelling is warm and tender with some reduction of movement in the adjacent joint. Osteosarcoma and chondrosarcoma rarely present with constitutional symptoms; Ewing's sarcoma, on the other hand, may give rise to malaise and pyrexia simulating osteomyelitis. Radiological appearance shows new bone formation alongside areas of bone destruction.

Ch 32, p. 429–30, *Fig 32.31, 32.32, 32.34*

15 The clinical features of rheumatoid arthritis are:

a – true, b – false, c – true, d – true, e – false

The clinical presentation and progress of affected joints in rheumatoid arthritis is variable depending on the severity of the inflammatory processes. Whilst the severe incapacity, joint laxity and joint deformities of advanced disease are characteristic, the earliest radiological change is a diffuse porosis of the involved bones with joint effusion.

Ch 36, p. 459, *Fig 36.13*

16 A positive Trendelenburg test:

a – true, b – false, c – false, d – false, e – true

The Trendelenburg test (sign) is positive when standing on one leg, the pelvis tilts down to the opposite side. This occurs in any condition that interferes with the action of the gluteus medius and minimus e.g.:

– gluteal paralysis or pain;
– congenital dislocation of the hip;
– fracture of the femoral neck;
– varus deformity of the femoral neck.

Ch 37, p. 463–4, *Fig 37.4*

17 In a patient complaining of pain and stiffness of the hip, the following observations assist in making a diagnosis:

a – true, b – true, c – true, d – true, e – false

Joint pain and/or stiffness produces a limp which is also a feature of limb shortening or muscle weakness. The Trendelenburg sign detects instability during standing and the Trendelenburg gait detects abductor muscle weakness. Limb shortening may be apparent or real; the former is produced by lumbosacral deformities, fixed flexion deformity or muscle spasm.

Ch 37, p. 463–6, *Fig 37.5, 37.6, 37.7, 37.8, 37.9*

18 A mother complained that her six-month-old infant has a lop-sided crawl and the legs do not open properly for nappy changes. An abnormal fold of skin is noticed over the thigh with apparent shortening of that limb. A diagnosis may be reached by:

a – false, b – true, c – true, d – true, e – true

Congenital dislocation of the hip should be detected during the neonatal clinical examination when most congenital anomalies come to light. Neurological examination excludes a palsy from an occult spinal anomaly. Failure to diagnose developmental hip dysplasia in infancy leads to irreducibility of the dislocation and an unstable gait with osteoarthritis supervening in early adult life.

Ch 37, p. 466, *Fig 37.10*

19 A healthy 10-year-old school girl complains of progressive pain in her hip and a limp for five months, she:

a – false, b – true, c – true, d – false, e – false

Perthes' disease and slipped upper femoral epiphysis produce ischaemic damage to the femoral head and are found between the ages of 5 and 15 years. There is pain on walking with a Trendelenburg gait and on examination there is a decreased range of joint movements. TB of the hip is uncommon and is secondary to primary disease in the lung or bowel. TB of the spine does not directly extend to the pelvis or the hip. Perthes' disease must be diagnosed early to forestall progressive deformity of the femoral head from weight bearing.

Ch 37, p. 467–8, *Fig 37.11, 37.12*

20   The clinical features associated with the diagnosis of a chronic slipped upper femoral epiphysis are:

a – true, b – true, c – false, d – true, e – true

In chronic slippage of the upper femoral epiphysis the epiphysis slips backward denuding the front of the femoral head where new bone is laid down when reduction is no longer possible. Pain associated with a limp is the usual symptom. There may be slight shortening with external rotation of the limb. Lateral plain radiology of the hip is usually diagnostic.

Ch 37, p. 468, *Fig 37.12*

21   The clinical findings of osteoarthritis of the hip are:

a – true, b – true, c – true, d – false, e – false

Hip pain is the predominant symptom of osteoarthritis which is worse on weight bearing. Joint stiffness leads to progressive restriction of all movements. There is a resultant limp (antalgic gait) with wasting of the hip muscles as the disease progresses. Characteristic radiological appearances are:

– distortion and subchondral sclerosis of the femoral head and acetabulum;
– osteophyte formation around joint margins;
– cyst formation;
– loss of joint space.

Ch 37, p. 468, *Fig 37.13*

22   In osteoarthritis of the knee:

a – true, b – false, c – true, d – true, e – true

Joint pain is the earliest symptom, which is worse after exercise. Stiffness follows inactivity with restriction of movements in advanced disease. Tenderness and crepitus or grating may be elicited on passive movement, and capsular thickening and effusion are detected on palpation. Plain radiology shows loss of joint space with subchondral sclerosis and osteophyte and cyst formation. Joint deformity with instability is found in advanced disease. Constitutional symptoms and extra-articular manifestations are uncommon.

Ch 37, p. 468, *Fig 37.13*
Ch 38, p. 473–4, *Fig 38.3, 38.4, 38.5, 38.6, 38.7, 38.8, 38.9*

23 A 59-year-old woman with a total hip replacement three years previously complains of pain in the groin radiating to the thigh resulting in a progressive limp. Diagnosis includes:

a – false, b – true, c – false, d – false, e – true

Long-term complications of prosthetic hip joints are common due to the frequency of this operation. Early complications are infective; there is usually a history of a wound infection which was slow to resolve following surgery. Delayed complications are due to malposition or loosening of the prosthesis; dislocation of the prosthesis or fracture of the femoral shaft around the prosthesis, usually resulting from a fall.

Ch 37, p. 469–70, *Fig 37.14*

24 The clinical findings in an adolescent with club foot are:

a – true, b – false, c – true, d – true, e – false

The recognition of club foot in infancy is necessary for early corrective measures. The condition may be bilateral or associated with congenital dislocation of the hip. The dorsum of the foot cannot be made to touch the shin as it can in the normal newborn.

Ch 40, p. 491–2, *Fig 40.1, 40.2, 40.3*

Self-assessment multiple choice question papers